SpringerBriefs in Public Health

Child Health

Series editor

Angelo P. Giardino, Houston, TX, USA

SpringerBriefs in Public Health present concise summaries of cutting-edge research and practical applications from across the entire field of public health, with contributions from medicine, bioethics, health economics, public policy, biostatistics, and sociology.

The focus of the series is to highlight current topics in public health of interest to a global audience, including health care policy; social determinants of health; health issues in developing countries; new research methods; chronic and infectious disease epidemics; and innovative health interventions.

Featuring compact volumes of 50 to 125 pages, the series covers a range of content from professional to academic. Possible volumes in the series may consist of timely reports of state-of-the art analytical techniques, reports from the field, snapshots of hot and/or emerging topics, elaborated theses, literature reviews, and in-depth case studies. Both solicited and unsolicited manuscripts are considered for publication in this series.

Briefs are published as part of Springer's eBook collection, with millions of users worldwide. In addition, Briefs are available for individual print and electronic purchase.

Briefs are characterized by fast, global electronic dissemination, standard publishing contracts, easy-to-use manuscript preparation and formatting guidelines, and expedited production schedules. We aim for publication 8–12 weeks after acceptance.

More information about this series at http://www.springer.com/series/11600

Janet Treadwell · Rebecca Perez
Debbie Stubbs · Jeanne W. McAllister
Susan Stern · Ruth Buzi

Case Management and Care Coordination

Supporting Children and Families
to Optimal Outcomes

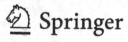

Janet Treadwell
Texas Children's Health Plan
Houston, TX
USA

Rebecca Perez
Carative Health Solutions
St Louis, MO
USA

Debbie Stubbs
Summit Reinsurance Services
Indianapolis, IN
USA

Jeanne W. McAllister
Pediatrics Children's Health Services
  Research Indiana University School
  of Medicine
Indianapolis, IN
USA

Susan Stern
URAC
Washington, DC
USA

Ruth Buzi
Baylor College of Medicine Teen Health
  Clinic
Houston, TX
USA

ISSN 2192-3698
ISBN 978-3-319-07223-4
DOI 10.1007/978-3-319-07224-1

ISSN 2192-3701 (electronic)
ISBN 978-3-319-07224-1 (eBook)

Library of Congress Control Number: 2014943931

Springer Cham Heidelberg New York Dordrecht London

Printed on acid-free paper

Springer is part of Springer Science+Business Media (www.springer.com)

Contents

Part I
Snapshot from the Field

Chapter 1
Process and Foundation

1.1 Growing Importance of Case Management and Care Coordination

The United States healthcare system poses risks and unnecessary expense due to fragmentation and lack of care coordination. Lack of communication, facilitation and planning for health care experiences can, at best, be confusing and at worst, fatal. One solution to weaving together necessary information with knowledge of best practice and consideration of individual preferences is care coordination. The Patient Protection and Affordable Care Act (PPACA) supports care coordination throughout descriptions of new models of care delivery and provisions for changes in quality arrived at through collaboration and coordination of care across all services and locations (PPACA 2010). Varying models of care coordination presented as components of health care reform system are in the process of testing and implementation. Change and modification will be in play as much more needs to be accomplished. The chapters of this text intend to increase awareness of care coordination and the role of the case manager in new and existing models of care. Families and healthcare professionals can benefit from understanding the professional role of the case manager, who possesses the skills and expertise to conduct and facilitate care coordination, which is integral to ensuring effective implementation of comprehensive care with its corollary improvements in efficiency and effectiveness. The importance of care coordination for children extends to the health of the family as described by Cousino and Hazen (2013) as well as Shudy et al. (2006), recognizing the physical and emotional stressors of being a family inclusive of a child with special healthcare needs.

This subject has relevance to children and families to equip them with an understanding of the definitions, key concepts, theory support, and structure of case management and care coordination. Knowledge of the benefits care coordination can provide to families is important in support of child health, family self-advocacy efforts, and for holding delivery models accountable to provide effective

© The Author(s) 2015
J. Treadwell et al., *Case Management and Care Coordination*,
SpringerBriefs in Child Health, DOI 10.1007/978-3-319-07224-1_1

care coordination as part of health benefit coverage. Practitioners will gain from this text, an improved understanding of care coordination, the role of case management, and suggested ways to implement effective features within the systems of care in which they practice. Discussion of the growing recognition and responsibilities of care coordination under new models of care delivery, leading to expectations and future direction is included.

1.2 Definitions and Differences

The use of the terms case management and care coordination as well as the roles of case managers, care managers, care coordinators, health coaches, and patient navigators pose confusion to both consumers and health care professionals. The Case Management Society of America (CMSA), which is a certification entity for professional case managers, posits the definition of case management as:

> "Case management is a collaborative process of assessment, planning, facilitation, care coordination, evaluation, and advocacy for options and services to meet an individual's and family's comprehensive health needs through communication and available resources to promote quality cost effective outcomes" (CMSA 2010).

Case managers are health care professionals who conduct the services and functions of case management and care coordination using knowledge of their specialty area combined with an understanding of the case management process. These individuals most frequently additionally hold licenses as registered nurses or social workers. Case managers may perform services independently or may hold a lead position in a care coordination team comprised of multiple people with varying roles and functions, focusing on a singular care plan of a child.

Care coordination is a responsibility of the entire healthcare delivery team. Communication and coordination with the child/family and all care providers delivering components of care to a child is both an ethical and professional responsibility of all health professionals caring for a child. There is an additional role of connection to the health care components from various sources, linking, where needed, to community and educational resources, and driving focus to the patient-centered plan of care. A case manager performs the oversight and connection of all activities to the benefit of the family and the provider team through care coordination.

The Agency for Healthcare Research and Quality (2007) defines care coordination as:

> "the deliberate organization of patient care activities between two or more participants (including the patient) involved in a patient's care to facilitate the appropriate delivery of health care services. Organizing care involves the marshaling of personnel and other resources needed to carry out all required patient care activities, and is often managed by the exchange of information among participants responsible for different aspects of care"
> Source: Closing the Quality Gap: A Critical Analysis of Quality Improvement Strategies (http://www.ahrq.gov/clinic/tp/caregaptp.htm).

Case managers (sometimes referred to as care managers) perform the functions of care coordination independently or as part of a team due to their expertise in facilitating care across the continuum. The most important part of care coordination is maintaining the client as the central focus of care while ensuring all other participants are duly involved and informed of needs of preferences of the client. This process eliminates duplication of services and connects the family to needed services for their child. Care coordination has gained recognition in importance over recent years. As an example, the promotion of effective communication and coordination of care is one of the National Quality Forum's six priorities, chosen due to their impact on health outcomes (National Quality Forum 2013). The American Nurses Association (2012) sites care coordination as a core professional standard and competency and the U.S. Department of Health and Human Services established the importance of care coordination in its' National Quality Strategy and the Institute of Medicine has gone on record with the assertion care coordination could save up to $240 billion in healthcare system savings (2010). The National Committee for Quality Assurance (NCQA) defines care coordination as a function that "supports information-sharing across providers, patients, types and levels of service, sites and time frames."

Family Tip: Access to a case manager or care coordination services may be offered by your health care provider or you may obtain case management and care coordination services by contacting the member services number on your health insurance card by asking for case management assistance.

Healthcare Professional Tip: Health care professionals can request case management services by contacting the individual's health plan and asking for an assessment.

1.3 The Case Management Process

The case management process gives case managers a structural approach to assisting individuals and families through the care and habilitation process for maximum outcome achievement. The process includes identification and selection of children who would benefit from program services, assessment and problem identification, development of a case management plan, implementation and coordination of the plan, evaluation of changes in the child's needs and progress, and follow-up to extend, modify, or close the plan. This is not a linear model as re-assessments and plan adjustments result from evaluations during the course of case management for the child. The term integrated case management explains a program approach that recognizes the interconnectedness of physical and behavioral health in developing an individualized plan of care for a child. From the perspective of a whole person/family, this approach recognizes one cannot separate the interplay between medical and emotional beings their environment, and their access to health services when developing a plan to identify needs and preferences that encompasses access, quality, safety, and efficiencies. Whether a diagnosis driven or integrated approach is used, managing complex health conditions occurs through use of evidence based guidelines and development of self-management strategies.

1.3.1 Identification and Selection

How does the case management team find a child needing services? Health care professionals are assessing for needs across all settings of care. Whether in the newborn nursery, during a well-child visit, or midst a hospitalization, identified needs trigger health care professionals that a child/family could benefit from care coordination support. Health care insurers identify children who for potential program inclusion by using analytic reporting on claim information. Pediatricians use developmental screening tools for proactive identification of children who might need care coordination and then refer to case managers for links to services. Screening tools can help in the assessment process. An example is the Child Adolescent Needs and Strengths (CANS) tool. The CANS captures parent/care-giver stress levels in addition to providing a resiliency picture of the child/adolescent. This is important to ensure the child and care giver(s) receive support and resources to achieve the highest level of functioning possible. Another screening tool is the Children with Special Healthcare Needs Screen which can identify areas needing further in-depth assessment (Table 1.1).

Programs for case management are most often considered voluntary. This means a request for participation is made to the child/family, explaining the available program and services as well as who will be interfacing with the family. Initial contact with a family is most often telephonic although may come in a face to face session or in written format. Care coordination staff asks for a verbal or written consent of participation from the responsible individual. Some health promotion or disease management programs are considered 'opt-out,' meaning that any person meeting the program inclusion criteria receives information and reminders or calls unless a person requests not to be included in a program.

1.3.2 Assessment

The initial assessment is extremely important however, can be time consuming. Expectations need to be set with families explaining the importance of this foundational activity. The individualized evaluation includes information that will outline future frequency, mode, and time of contacts and is inclusive of defining cultural and religious preferences, literacy screening, and assessment of barriers to function and treatment engagement. The goal is to obtain a comprehensive and accurate baseline describing the child across a holistic set of domains.

Table 1.1 Tools used for pediatric assessment of special healthcare needs

Child adolescent needs and strengths (CANS): http://www.dhs.state.or.us/caf/safety_model/procedure_manual/ch04/ch4-section6.pdf
CSHCN screener: http://www.childhealthdata.org/docs/cshcn/cshcn-screener-cahmi-quickguide-pdf.pdf
Parents' evaluation of developmental status (PEDS): http://www.Pedstest.com
Modified checklist for autism in toddlers (MCHAT): http://www.mchatscreen.com
Ages and Stages Questionnaires (ASQ): http://agesandstages.com/

Table 1.2 Domains of assessment

Physiology	Environmental
Psychosocial	Health behaviors
Spiritual	Self-care

The initial assessment is perhaps the most essential part of the process as it is extremely comprehensive and begins establishing the relationship of trust integral to optimal success. Assessment information is gained from a variety of sources including the child/family, current health care providers, records of past health care experiences, school educational plans (if applicable) and assessment of the community offerings of available services. Items included in the assessment cover domains inclusive of medical and psychosocial areas that best describe an individual in relation to their environment as well as questions to gauge specific needs and preferences of the child/family that may arise from cultural or spiritual beliefs (Table 1.2). The assessment does take some time so can be broken down into more than one session as needed to support family comfort (Table 1.3). Supplementing the assessment information are screening tools which may be initiated by the case manager, a primary care physician, or specialist.

1.3.3 Problem Identification and Care Plan Development

The assessment information results are shared in a care planning session with the child/family creating clinical (medical/behavioral), social service, and wellness goals. Inclusion of the medical/behavioral home practitioners optimally occurs in real time or through communication by care coordination staff to create a shared care plan that is given to the child/family, the primary practitioner, and specialists or ancillary care providers as applicable. The team-created care plan creates a unified document to support coordination and consistency for service and to reach the child's goals.

The National Initiative for Children's Healthcare Quality and the Center for Medical Home Improvement held a working collaborative to develop contents and

Table 1.3 Contents of typical assessment

Assessment of clients' health status, including condition-specific issues
Documentation of clinical history, including medications
Initial assessment of the activities of daily living
Initial assessment of mental health status, including cognitive functions
Initial assessment of life-planning activities
Evaluation of cultural and linguistic needs, preferences or limitations
Evaluation of visual and hearing needs, preferences or limitations
Evaluation of caregiver resources and involvement
Evaluation of available benefits within the organization and from community resources
Development of an individualized case management case management plan, including prioritized goals, that considers the clients' and caregivers' goals, preferences and desired level of involvement in the case management plan
Identification of barriers to meeting goals or complying with the plan
Facilitation of member referrals to resources and follow-up on process to determine whether the member acts on the referral
Development of a schedule for follow-up communication with clients
Development and communication of member self-management plans for clients
A process to assess progress against case management plans for clients

explanation of a comprehensive care plan for children with special healthcare needs (http://www.medicalhomeinfo.org/downloads/pdfs/ComprehensiveCarePlanning. pdf). The document contains sample forms with topical areas of importance, stressing the need for a plan of care whether in paper copy format, contained on a memory stick or accessible through the internet.

> Family Tip: Families are to be included in care plan development. It is important that your family's needs and preferences are included in the document. Ask for a copy of your child's care plan and ask that revisions be made when your child's health condition changes.

> Health Care Professional Tip: To improve compliance with your instructions for medication, treatment and testing, share those items with the case manager to improve continuity and outcomes. The goal is use of a shared electronic care plan enabling all practitioners to see and interact with the child/family in one document.

1.3.4 Implementation and Coordination

A care coordination team member employs a process of implementing activities to address barriers and prioritized goals as well as performs ongoing assessment and documentation to monitor the quality of care and services provided. During interim evaluation of the care plan, the case manager adjusts interventions based upon information drawn from the child/family and all care providers to ensure

Table 1.4 Goal evaluation measures of patient-centered plan

Goal achievement
Adherence to medication/treatment regimen(s)
Barriers to compliance with provider appointments
Development of self-management skills
Ability of child/family recognition of signs and symptoms of worsening chronic condition
Nutritional and cognitive status
Psychosocial adjustments
Satisfaction with current services (equipment, professional)
Adequacy of school provision to meet needs
Understanding of emergency/disaster plan
Evaluation of results of education provision related to health and care access
Need for home visits for education or resource application
Consideration of transition needs
Existing support and communication between child/family and providers
Achieved links in the community setting

goals are addressed. Case managers review and update care plans as needed based on condition changes but no less frequently than on a semi-annual basis (see Table 1.4).

1.3.5 Evaluation and Follow Up

Engagement with the child/family is an ongoing process that enables the coordination team to perform reassessments and develop measurement of the child's progress in achieving current and prioritized goals. Evaluation assesses movement outlined in the plan of care and determines the impact of care coordination and care interventions on outcomes (Table 1.5). The case manager establishes, measurable case management goals, which promote evaluation of the access, cost and quality of the care provided to the child to facilitate measures of goal achievement that directly result from the case management interventions.

Reliable outcome data can serve as a basis of impact to future practice. Case managers use their goal directed patient- centered practice to not only evaluate each individual to monitor but the overall program they are delivering on a population management basis identifying patterns to maximize clinically positive, cost-effective outcomes. This program evaluation includes aggregate reporting of health outcomes, satisfaction surveys of families, cost analysis, and notes contact rate, frequency and care plan revisions. Outcomes are frequently then compared to national benchmarks such as the Kids Inpatient Database (http://www.hcup-us. ahrq.gov/kidoverview.jsp) or the Centers for Disease Control and Prevention Chronic Disease Calculator (2009).

Table 1.5 Resources for family centered coordination approach

Teamwork and communication module PS 103 http://app.ihi.org/lms/coursedetailview.aspx?CourseGUID=3e37eb4a-4928-4d8b-976e-3a2a1a 5f2c08&CatalogGUID=6cb1c614-884b-43ef-9abd-d90849f183d4
Patient and Family Centered Care PFC 101 http://app.ihi.org/lms/coursedetailview.aspx?CourseGUID=8eb52137-21d7-4b30-afcd-fd781 de6d6d5&CatalogGUID=6cb1c614-884b-43ef-9abd-d90849f183d4
Writing the IFSP: National dissemination center for children with disabilities http://ifspweb.org/
Tools to foster the collaboration with patient and family advisors http://www.ipfcc.org/tools/downloads-tools.html

1.3.5.1 Case Closure Criteria

Care coordination needs may resolve in situations that are time-limited or where self-management skills progress to a level of independence. Case closure may also occur due to change in insurance coverage, or due to aging into an adult system of healthcare delivery. Closure of the coordinating relationship may terminate due to a child's death or to child/family refusal to initiate or continue with services. The case manager documents the rationale for case closure as well as documentation of status at the time of close as a child may return to need services due to an exacerbation of condition or change of coverage.

1.4 Theories and Models of Practice for Case Management and Care Coordination

Care coordination has value for transition across services and as an organizing framework to support best practice. It is especially significant when addressing needs of children with multiple chronic conditions. According to a white paper published by the Partnership to Fight Chronic Disease, one in fifteen children in the United States has a chronic disease (Thorpe 2013).

Care coordination addresses the need for education and support of families through alignment of both treatment and communication using the structure of an evidenced-based model. In addition to elements of professional education and health system knowledge, case managers use theory and evidence-based practice to support families across the continuum of care.

Fig. 1.1 Wagner, EH.
Chronic Disease
Management: What Will It
Take to Improve Care for
Chronic Illness? Effective
Clinical Practice. 1998;1:2–4

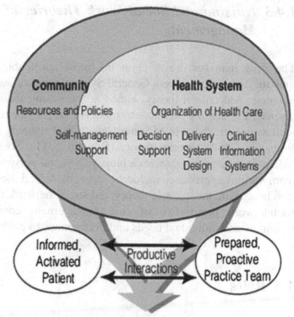

Community

Resources and Policies

Self-management
Support

Health System

Organization of Health Care

Decision   Delivery   Clinical
Support   System   Information
           Design   Systems

Informed,
Activated
Patient

Productive
Interactions

Prepared,
Proactive
Practice Team

Functional and Clinical Outcomes

1.4.1 The Chronic Care Model

Wagner's Chronic Care Model (Fig. 1.1) supports an informed and activated patient (child/family) coupled with a prepared and proactive practice team. The model also acknowledges the influences of the community and the healthcare system on ultimate patient outcomes which is an important part of coordinating across school standards, neighborhood and state resources as well as navigating the health system for access and necessary services. Wagner's model is advocated in medical home models and has evidence of improved delivery of care to recipients when adopted by practitioners (Coleman et al. 2009).

1.4.2 Continuum of Healthcare Model

The Case Management Society of America (CMSA) supports a continuum model of health care. Focusing on a patient centered model of case management delivery, the case management process is viewed within a circular model of financial, ethical and legal, social support and care providers. The philosophy targets optimum client wellness and function through communication, advocacy, education, resource identification, and facilitation of services to benefit the client, support system, healthcare delivery system and reimbursement (CMSA Standards of Practice for Case Management 2010).

1.4.3   Nursing and Social Work Theories of Case Management

The case manager draws upon the most applicable theories to apply to any modality/specialty of need. General System's theory, exploring relationships in the universe, and critical theory, aimed at translating theory into practice, have been discussed in nursing literature as models to represent case management practice as well as nursing theories of Sister Calista Roy's theory of adaptation, and Dr. Jean Watson's Caring Science theory (Roussel 2011). Social work theory supporting case management emphasizes a biopsychosocial perspective combining knowledge from various approaches including strengths-based theory, use of learning theory, psychoanalytic theory, role theory and social network theory (Brandell 2010). The social work perspective of case management combines theory, community resources and individual needs and preferences to enable optimal clinical practice.

1.5   Roles

Depending on the program, diagnosis of a child, and employer of the case manager, roles may vary. The CMSA Standards of Practice describe the role of the case manager, use of evidence-based guidelines in practice, the role of minimizing fragmentation, navigating transitions of care, incorporating adherence guidelines and other standardized practice tools, expanding the interprofessional team in planning care for individuals, and improving patient safety. Another professional case management organization that focuses primarily on hospital case management, the American Case Management Association, adds the element of resource utilization into the role of case management through their Standards of Practice indicating the case manager:

> "assures prudent utilization of all resources (fiscal, human, environmental, equipment and services) by evaluating the resources available to the patient and balancing cost and quality to ensure the optimal clinical and financial outcomes (2013)."

The team approach to care coordination has as the most important member, the child/family. Case managers lead the care coordination teams due to their professional experience in assessment and collaboration. The team also may include: registered nurses, social workers, experienced parent partners, community health workers, educational specialists, and often dieticians in addition to the primary care medical home (pediatrician) and specialist healthcare professionals. Interprofessional collaboration defines the supporting culture of the care coordination team. The emphasis is on clear communication, professional accountability, shared decision making, and mutual trust across all roles on the team to result in cooperative interaction achieving improved outcomes from teamwork as opposed to a singular practitioner approach (McDonald et al. 2007).

Family Tip: The parent-to-parent model, using people who have experienced care of a child with complex health needs, is increasingly being applied in health care systems across the United States and is considered a true measure and best practice of Medical Home for Children and Youth with Special Health Care Needs (CYSHCN).

Team members conducting care coordination provide a contribution to the individuals served and to overall population health as the team scope includes the triple aim of improving the quality and experience of care as well as overall cost through developing efficiency and effectiveness through coordination (http://www.ihi.org/offerings/Initiatives/TripleAim/Pages/default.aspx). The team approach requires valuing the opinions and experience of the patient/family and other team members. The goal being to effectively communicate pertinent clinical information and treatment preferences across all professional types and organize that care to avoid duplication, support safe transfers and care transitions involved in the child's care, extending to the school and community setting as needed. Use of evidence based guidelines delivers consistency across team members and sets expectations with the family, essential when managing complex health conditions. Team training in guidelines as well as resources and culture build is necessary (Table 1.5). Care coordination requires interaction among all roles as each person on the team has a unique expertise to add to the child's success and resiliency build.

Family Tip: Movement in prioritized goals is to be addressed during each contact. The case coordination team member should create a shared expectation of communication frequency and type with the child/family/practitioner to discuss case management strategies and adjustments in the plan of care. Ask for the "who, when, and what" of contact as well as numbers to call in case of questions and emergencies.

Care Professional Tip: Team coordination supports access of families to informed professionals without repeating details of their child's information. Developing teams with shared understanding of prioritizes goals to deliver seamless coordination improves satisfaction of the care coordination team as well as families.

1.6 Ethics

Members of the care coordination team have an obligation to behave in a moral and ethical manner. Professionals are responsible to a code of professional conduct (nursing, social work, etc.) and team members responsible to ethical standards of their affiliated employer. Included in the concept of ethical practice and training for care coordination teams are the areas of: confidentiality, client respect, cultural competency, disclosure of conflicts of interest, and acknowledgement of self-determination. The principles of beneficence, nonmalfeasance, autonomy (respecting right to choose), and justice and fidelity (follow through) are core to care coordination practice (http://ccmcertification.org/sites/default/files/downloads/2012/41%20-%20Ethics%20issue%20brief.pdf). Ethical considerations underscore the primary obligation to the child. Conflicts can arise for the case manager or care coordination team member due to issues of benefits, policies or regulations that require an ethical evaluation by the administrative team.

In promoting self-advocacy, the care coordination team supports family-based decision-making and self-management by providing education and promoting shared decision making across the care team. The care coordination team is responsible for advocating on behalf of the child, facilitating access, needed services, and addressing barriers/disparities that may occur during care coordination (http://www.preventioninstitute.org/tools/focus-area-tools/health-equity-toolkit.html).

Family Tip: If you feel that a bias or obstruction to needed care is present, ask for a review/appeal of your case by management staff of the entity supplying care coordination services, requesting an ethics review.

Healthcare Professional Tip: Be familiar with the Code of Ethics of your licensed profession as well as your employer. Reveal any conflicts of interest which may arise to your employer.

References

Agency for Healthcare Research and Quality. (2007). *Closing the quality gap: A critical analysis of quality improvement strategies*. Publication No. 04(07)-0051-7. Rockville, MD. Retrieved from http://www.ahrq.gov/clinic/tp/caregaptp.htm.

American Case Management Association. (2013). *Standards of practice and scope of services for hospital/health system case management*. American Case Management Association, Little Rock, AR. Retrieved from http://www.acmaweb.org/section.asp?sID=22.

American Nurses Association. (2012, June) *The value of nursing care coordination*. Retrieved from: http://www.nursingworld.org/carecoordinationwhitepaper.

Brandell, J. (Ed.). (2010). *Theory and practice of clinical social work*, (2nd ed.). New York: Columbia University Press.

Case Management Society of America. (2010). *Standards of practice*. Retrieved from http://www.cmsa.org/Individual/MemberResources/StandardsofPracticeforCaseManagement/tabid/69/Default.aspx.

Center for Disease Control and Prevention. *Chronic disease calculator*. Retrieved at http://www.cdc.gov/chronicdisease/resources/calculator/index.htm.

Coleman, K., Austin, B., Brach, C., & Wagner, E. (2009). Evidence on the chronic care model in the new millennium. *Health Affairs, 28*(1), 75–85.

Cousino, M., & Hazen, R. (2013). Parenting stress among caregivers of children with chronic illness: A systematic review. *Journal of Pediatric Psychology, 38*(8), 809–828. doi:10.1093/jpepsy/jst049.

Healthcare Cost and Utilization Project. *Kids Inpatient database*. Retrieved from http://www.hcup-us.ahrq.gov/kidoverview.jsp.

Institute of Medicine. (2010). *Roundtable on value and science driven health care: The healthcare imperative: lowering costs and improving outcomes. Workshop Series Summary*. Washington, DC: National Academic Press. 2010.

Institute for Healthcare Improvement. *IHI triple aim initiative*. Retrieved from http://www.ihi.org/offerings/Initiatives/TripleAim/Pages/default.aspx.

McDonald, K., Sundram, V., Bravata, D., Lewis, R., Lin, N., Kraft, S., McKinnon, M., Paguntalan, H., & Owens, D. (2007, June). *Care coordination. AHRQ Publication No. 04(07)-0051-7.* Rockville, MD: Agency for Healthcare Research and Quality.

National Quality Forum, Prioritization Measures, September 16, 2013, Retrieved from: NQF.org.

Patient Protection and Affordable Care Act. (2010). Pub Law No. 111–148.

Roussel, L. (2011). *Management and Leadership for nurse administrators*, (6th Edn.). Burlington, MA: Jones and Bartlett,

Shudy, M., Lihinie de Almeida, M., Ly, S., Landon, C., Groft, S., Jenkins, T., & Nicholson, C. (2006, December). Impact of pediatric critical illness and injury on families: a systematic literature review. *Pediatrics, 118*, S203–S218. doi: 10.1542/peds.2006-0951B.

Thorpe, J. (2013, April). Needs great evidence lacking. *Partnership to Fight Chronic Disease.* Retrieved from http://www.scribd.com/doc/137602733/Needs-Great-Evidence-Lacking-White-Paper.

Wagner, E. (1998). Chronic disease management: What will it take to improve care for chronic illness? *Effective Clinical Practice, 1*, 2–4.

Chapter 2
Essential Skills for Case Managers

2.1 Essential Skill Overview

If you ask ten people what case management means to them, you will most likely get ten different answers. Though case management has been around since the late 70s, there has not been a clear understanding of the role. There may be several reasons for the lack of clarity. The practice of case management extends across all health care settings, including payer, provider, government, employer, community, and home environment. The practice also varies in degrees of complexity and comprehensiveness based on the setting, health conditions, reimbursement, and healthcare profession (Powell and Tahan 2008).

Since the enactment of the Health Maintenance Organization Act of 1973, case managers have been working to develop and define the role. The work of the Case Management Society of America (CMSA) has been instrumental in the development and standardization of the practice of case management. Founded in 1990, CMSA (www.cmsa.org) is the leading non-profit association dedicated to the support and development of case management. The CMSA developed Standards of Practice that utilize the essential skills of case managers to provide a foundation for all case managers, regardless of practice setting. The standards were first published in 1995 and revised in 2002 and 2010. The majority of case management programs today are based on the CMSA standards (http://www.cmsa.org/portals/0/pdf/memberonly/StandardsOfPractice.pdf).

The case manager performs the primary functions of assessment, planning, facilitation and advocacy, which are achieved through collaboration with the patient and other health care professionals involved in the patient's care. Key responsibilities of case management have been identified by nationally recognized professional societies and certifying bodies through case management roles and functions research. When asked to describe the essential skills necessary for an effective case manager, it was best to work from the CMSA standards of practice

© The Author(s) 2015
J. Treadwell et al., *Case Management and Care Coordination*,
SpringerBriefs in Child Health, DOI 10.1007/978-3-319-07224-1_2

which really are the "gold standards" for case management. This chapter will discuss how case managers use specific skills within their practice to achieve standards of practice. Twelve standards will be used to example essential case management skills.

The CMSA guiding principles for case management include:

- Using a patient-centric, collaborative partnership approach.
- Facilitating self-determination and self-care through the tenets of advocacy, shared decision making and education.
- Using a comprehensive, holistic approach.
- Practicing cultural competence with awareness and respect for diversity.
- Promoting the use of evidence-based care.
- Promoting optimal patient safety.
- Promoting the integration of behavioral change science and principles.
- Linking with community resources.
- Assisting with navigating the health care system to achieve successful care, for example during transitions.
- Pursuing professional excellence and maintain competence in practice.
- Promoting quality outcomes and measurement of those outcomes.
- Supporting and maintaining compliance with federal, state, local, organizational, and certification rules and regulations CMSA (2010) Standards of Practice for Case Management.

As you look at the guiding principles it is easy to see that a professional case manager who can facilitate these operations must have a basic set of skills in addition to their foundational healthcare license. For example, using a patient-centered approach is apart from the traditional model of health care. Case managers have collaboration as an essential skill as they come from a place of no formal authority to shale relationships and actions of children/families and their care providers. Another important skill set is cultural competency and use of reflective practice. Knowing that the family are the ultimate decision makers in care decisions and practices translates to a required skill set impacting a case manager's approach to families and use of education, self-management tools, and shared -decision making. An effective case manager realizes they are dealing with individuals with different value systems, cultural beliefs, and socioeconomic backgrounds. There are generally no negative consequences for non-adherence to a plan of care other than recurrent signs and symptoms of the underlying disease. The effectiveness of a case manager really stems from an individual who is truly passionate about what they do and knows how to communicate with patients and support systems in a way in which they can fully understand their diagnosis, treatment expectations, desired outcomes, and consequences for non-adherence.

2.2 Standard #1: Patient Selection Process for Case Management

The case manager should identify and select patients who can most benefit from case management services available in a particular practice setting.

Not everyone needs or wants case management. Most programs use some form of high-risk screening criteria to assess for inclusion in case management programs. The screening criteria generally include medical and psychosocial considerations such as chronic, catastrophic, or terminal illness; social issues such as a history of abuse, neglect, no known social support, or lives alone; repeated admissions; and financial issues. The essential skill for the case manager is a strong clinical background to understand the severity of a child's clinical condition combined with a proficient use of analytic tools that help identify risks and priorities.

Tips for Parents: Try to identify barriers to care/adherence and whether a case manager may be helpful in decreasing or eliminating the barriers to improve outcomes.

Tips for Healthcare Professionals: Case managers generally have the additional time to spend with patients and support systems to perform a comprehensive assessment of a situation and help identify barriers to care/adherence. In the situation where a case manager has a complex patient or situation, a referral to a case manager for initial screening may be beneficial.

2.3 Standard #2: Patient Assessment

The case manager should complete a health and psychosocial assessment, taking into account the cultural and linguistic needs of each patient.

This is a very important step in the case management process and it may take several conversations with the child/family, and providers to get a comprehensive picture of the care needs and barriers. A good case manager is able to ask the right questions to get to the heart of an issue. Sources of information can include patient/support systems interviews, healthcare provider discussions, medical records, claims data, and utilization history. The information included in the assessment may vary depending on the reason for the case management referral but generally include physical, psychosocial, and functional components. Caregiver support is very important for patients unable to provide self-care. Case managers as educators can present information in an understandable was, noting the health literacy level of families, to make sure families are able to participate as informed consumers understanding their choices in care decisions.

2.4 Standard #3: Problem Opportunity/Identification

The case manager should identify problems or opportunities that would benefit from case management intervention.

The most important point to make is that the patient/support systems are in agreement regarding the problems/opportunities identified. If the patient does not consider a certain behavior a "problem" he/she will see no reason to change the behavior. If the patient in engaging in harmful behavior but is not willing to recognize the behavior as harmful or change it, the role of the healthcare provider is to educate the patient regarding the potential negative consequences of that behavior and hopefully revisit it in future interactions. The essential skill for assessment is the communication technique of motivational interviewing which supports families in considering their options and opportunities to achieve desired goals.

2.5 Standard #4: Planning

The case manager should identify immediate, short-term, long-term, and ongoing needs, as well as develop appropriate and necessary case management strategies and goals to address those needs.

The patient/support systems must be involved in the plan of care and patient preferences and desires have to be incorporated. There is not "one size fits all" plan of care. Customizing the plan to meets the needs of the patient is a key component to adherence. Case managers incorporate the essential skill of organization, much as a project manager would move through any given assignment. The case management process gives them a framework to follow to check milestones and organize their process.

> Tips for Parents: Make your preferences and needs known during the planning stage. The goals must be reasonable and achievable and parental/caregiver input matters!

> Tips for Healthcare Providers: Be sure the goals are objective and measureable. Use of SMART goals is recommended:

Specific
Measureable
Attainable
Realistic
Timely

(Doran 1981).

2.6 Standard #5: Monitoring

The case manager should employ ongoing assessment and documentation to measure the patient's response to the plan of care.

Once the plan of care has been outlined, the case manager will monitor the progress of the patient towards the desired outcomes. Having SMART goals makes the process of monitoring easier. During this process, the case manager may also serve as an educator and coach, facilitating movement toward desired outcomes. Ultimately the patient/support systems are responsible for adherence to the plan of care, but they may need the guidance and encouragement along the way. The case manager will document ongoing collaboration with the patient, support systems or caregiver, providers, and other pertinent stakeholders, so that the patient's response to interventions is reviewed and incorporated into the plan of care.

Changing behaviors can be difficult especially when habits have been formed. As mentioned previously, case managers cannot make anyone do anything. People generally will not make changes unless they realize a significant benefit and are ready to try. One of tools used to determine a patient's readiness to change is motivational interviewing (http://pharmacy.auburn.edu/barkebn/Resume/Teaching %20Motivational%20Interviewing%20with%20a%20Virtual%20Patient.htm) (Auburn University Motivational Training Institute 2009).

Once again you see the skill of motivational interviewing (MI) as an important approach to improving adherence first reported in the addiction literature (Rollnick et al. 2008). It is a process used to determine readiness to engage in a target behavior (e.g. taking a medicine as prescribed) in order to apply specific verbal skills and strategies based upon the patient's level of readiness. MI increases treatment adherence by stimulating or enhancing the patient's intrinsic motivation in order to address and resolve ambivalence and resistance (major barriers to adherence) rather than by providing extrinsic motivation in the form of arguments, advice, and orders.

Monitoring will include verification that the plan of care continues to be appropriate, realistic, understood, accepted by the child/family and supported by the care team. The plan of care may need to be revised due to changes in the patient's condition, lack of response to the care plan, preference changes, transitions across settings, and newly identified barriers to care and services. An effective case manager realizes things may not always go as planned and will have recommendations for alternative plans of care.

Tips for Parents: Ask yourself, "do I really think there is a problem with my child and am I willing to commitment to making the necessary changes to improve adherence?"

2.7 Standard #6: Outcomes

The case manager should maximize the patient's health, wellness, safety, adaptation, and self-care through quality case management, patient satisfaction, and cost-efficiency.

Case mangers work with patients and support systems to provide support and guidance which hopefully results in achieving the outcomes outlined in the plan of care. Case management is an outcome driven process that is time limited. The expectation is the child/family, as possible, will ultimately take full responsibility for adhering to the plan of care independent from the case manager. The essential skill of collaboration is put into place when maximizing recovery through connection to community resources, facilitating integration at school and in other areas of interest to the child such as sport opportunities. The concept of self-care should be stressed from the very beginning and throughout the case management process. If the patient is unable to engage in self-care, the case manager will work to offer suggestions for caregivers and alternative support systems.

2.8 Standard #7: Termination of Case Management Services

The case manager should appropriately terminate case management services based upon established case closure guidelines.

These guidelines may differ in various case management practice settings. As stated earlier, case management is time limited process with the expectation that the patient will become independent in adhering to the plan of care.

However, sometimes there is the necessity to support families through a case where the opportunities for self-management will not be possible. The essential skill of life care planning incorporates a range of service the case manager can support focusing on what will be the required needs of the individual throughout their life course to support them in meeting their goals.

An effective case manager maintains open communication with patients and healthcare providers regarding the potential termination of case management services well before services are terminated. Patients and healthcare providers should feel comfortable with the termination of services and confident that the patient can do it independently.

2.9 Standard #8: Facilitation, Coordination, and Collaboration

The case manager should facilitate coordination, communication, and collabo-ration with the patient and other stakeholders in order to achieve goals and maximize positive patient outcomes.

The healthcare system is complex and sometimes hard to navigate. Case managers can be instrumental in developing proactive, patient-centered relation-ships and communication with the patient, and other necessary stakeholders to maximize outcomes. Patients may see several healthcare providers and obtain care from a variety of facilities. Communication between providers may be minimal or non-existent, with no single entity providing oversight for the plan of care. The case manager may become instrumental in collaborating with the various entities to ensure that all parties are aware of the plan of care that has taken into con-sideration the personal preferences of the patient.

An essential skill for an effective case manager is the ability to negotiate; to reconcile potentially differing points of view. Not everyone sees things the same way which can sometimes the biggest barrier to developing the plan of care. The role of the case manager includes clearly communicating the pros and cons of a treatment plan. Laying all of the cards on the table so patients can make a fully informed decision regarding what they want to do moving forward.

2.10 Standard #9: Qualifications for Case Managers

Case managers should maintain competence in their area(s) of practice by having one of the following:

1. *Current, active, and unrestricted licensure or certification in a health or human services discipline that allows the professional to conduct an assessment independently as permitted within the scope of practice of the discipline; and/ or*
2. *Baccalaureate or graduate degree in social work, nursing, or another health or human services field that promotes the physical, psychosocial, and/or voca-tional well-being of the persons being served. The degree must be from an institution that is fully accredited by a nationally recognized educational accreditation organization, and the individual must have completed a super-vised field experience in case management, health, or behavioral health as part of the degree requirements.*

There are people in a variety of settings, with a variety of experiences and education, holding the title of case manager. The interventions provided vary greatly based on the patient population and practice setting. It is also important maintain compliance with national and/or local laws and regulations that apply to the jurisdictions(s) and discipline(s) in which the case manager practices. Healthcare is an ever changing field which requires case managers to maintain competence through relevant and ongoing continuing education, study, and consultation. Most importantly, a case manager must practice within their area(s) of expertise, making timely and appropriate referrals to, and seeking consultation with, others when needed.

Tips for Parents: When working with a case manager, inquire about their credentials, educational background, and experience.

2.11 Standard #10: Legal

The case manager should adhere to applicable local, state, and federal laws, as well as employer policies, governing all aspects of case management practice, including patient privacy and confidentiality rights. It is the responsibility of the case manager to work within the scope of his/her licensure.

This standard is broken down into two main areas, Confidentiality/Patient Privacy and Consent for Case management.

2.11.1 Confidentiality and Patient Privacy

The case manager should adhere to applicable local, state, and federal laws, as well as employer policies, governing the patient, patient privacy, and confidentiality rights and act in a manner consistent with the patient's best interest.

Privacy laws do change and it is the responsibility of the case manager to maintain up-to-date knowledge of, and adherence to, applicable laws and regulations concerning confidentiality, privacy, and protection of client medical information issues.

Maintaining confidentiality of protected health information (PHI) is an important part of the case manager's practice. Case managers work closely with patients and support systems and often collect information that is highly sensitive. Case managers must remember they cannot share patient specific information with other individuals without the consent of the patient.

2.11.2 Consent for Case Management Services

The case manager should obtain appropriate and informed patient consent before case management services are implemented.

Patients need to be actively involved in the plan of care for adherence to occur. Getting the patient's consent to engage in the case management process is the first step towards obtaining some level of commitment by the patient. Patients need to understand the role and objectives of a case manager which should be shared prior to obtaining patient consent. Sharing this information allows the patient to make an informed consent. There should be some evidence that the patient and support systems where thoroughly informed of the following:

- Proposed case management process and services relating to the patient's health conditions and needs
- Possible benefits and costs of such services
- Alternatives to the proposed services
- Potential risks and consequences of the proposed services and alternatives
- Client's right to refuse the proposed case management services, and potential risks and consequences related to such refusal

An effective case manager validates throughout the process that the patient is the "driver" of the plan of care with the expectation that the case manager will decrease their involvement as the patient works toward self-efficacy.

2.12   Standard #12: Advocacy

The case manager should advocate for the patient at the service-delivery, benefits-administration, and policy-making levels.

Navigating the healthcare system can be confusing and complex. Case managers are instrumental in facilitating access to necessary and appropriate services while educating the patient and support systems about resource availability within practice settings and the community. Case managers promote patient self-determination, informed and shared decision-making, autonomy, and self-advocacy. Case managers identify the needs, strengths, and goals of the patient and incorporate this information into the plan of care. Case managers recognize and try to eliminate disparities in accessing high quality care. Such disparities may be related to race, ethnicity, national origin, sex, sexual orientation, age, religion, political beliefs, physical, mental, or cognitive disability.

2.13   Standard #13: Cultural Competency

The case manager should be aware of, and responsive to, cultural and demographic diversity of the population and specific patient profiles.

People come from different countries, hold different beliefs, and embraced a variety of cultural norms. Cultural differences need to be incorporated into the plan of care to enhance adherence. An effective case manager understands relevant cultural information and communicates effectively, respectfully, and sensitively within the patient's cultural context. Language barriers may also be instrumental in adherence. Assessment of patient's linguistic needs and identifying resources to enhance proper communication is very important. Patients cannot adhere to a plan of care if they are unable to understand what is expected of them. Case managers may need to use an interpreter and written materials in the appropriate language. An understanding of cultural communication patterns of speech volume, context, tone, kinetics, space, and other similar verbal/nonverbal communication patterns can be helpful.

References

Auburn University Motivational Training Institute. 4–6 Dec 2009.

Case Management Society of America. Case management adherence guidelines. Retrieved from http://www.cmsa.org/CMAG.

CMSA. (2010). Standards of practice for case management. Retrieved from http://www.cmsa.org/Individual/MemberToolkit/StandardsofPractice/tabid/69/Default.aspx.

Doran, G. T. (1981). There's a S.M.A.R.T. way to write management's goals and objectives. *Management Review*, *70*(11), 35–36. Retrieved from http://www.ncdhhs.gov/humanresources/pms/pm/smart.pdf.

Powell, S. K., & Tahan, H. A. (2008). *CMSA core curriculum for case management* (2nd ed.). Philadelphia, PA: Lippincott Williams & Wilkins.

Rollnick, S., Miller, W., & Butler, C. (2008). *Motivational interviewing in health care*. New York, NY: Guilford Press.

Chapter 3
Integrated Case Management

3.1 Definition and Background

3.1.1 Overview

Health professionals must have a multidimensional approach for patients with complex health conditions to regain stable health and function. Integrated Case Management is a highly personalized approach which addresses all segments of the health system, medical issues, behavioral issues, and social barriers. Current problems related to care of the complex patient result from fragmented communications and equally fragmented coordination of medical and behavioral conditions, and perhaps the presence of multiple chronic conditions (Chen et al. 2012). The Agency for Healthcare Quality and Research (AHRQ) defines a complex patient as a person with two or more active conditions (Chen et al. 2012). *The Integrated Case Management Manual: Assisting Complex Patients Regain Physical and Mental Health* defines complexity as the presence of concurrent medical and behavioral conditions, multiple chronic illnesses, social barriers, and/or noncommunicating segments of health system (Kathol 2010).

3.1.2 Complexity

Complexity occurs when one chronic condition effects the treatment or outcomes of another chronic condition, recognizing the burden of one condition may be greater than another. Complexity not only affects the potential for stability of the patient, but also effects families and caregivers psychologically, socially and financially. Adults with complex conditions have a unique set of challenges, but the pediatric patient with complex conditions can test the abilities of even the most seasoned health professional.

© The Author(s) 2015
J. Treadwell et al., *Case Management and Care Coordination*,
SpringerBriefs in Child Health, DOI 10.1007/978-3-319-07224-1_3

Children with complex conditions are often seen by multiple providers. Fragmented interaction among these providers leads to inconsistent and poorly managed care (Chen et al. 2012). The needs of patients with chronic conditions are not adequately met by the acute care system; they require a defined management plan that includes regular assessment, defined interventions, and well coordinated communication among patients, caregivers and the primary care team (Chen et al. 2012).

Integrated Pediatric Case Management is a relatively new concept, but the well-established foundation of adult integrated case management can be adapted to meet the needs of children and youth with complex conditions (Kathol 2010). Children and youth with complex health conditions are just as likely to experience treatment resistance, symptom persistence, social impairment and high healthcare utilization as the complex adult patient (Kathol 2010). And while there are additional considerations when working with the pediatric population, addressing all barriers to improvement is expected to result in overall progress. When working with pediatric patients with health complexity, additional considerations include the health of the family or caregiver, the child's attendance and performance in school, which is available to provide assistance and additional support, and whether the child has a safe and nurturing environment. These issues are of equal value to the child's medical or psychological conditions as they cannot be adequately managed without appropriate support and safety. The parent or caregiver of the complex pediatric patient may also need case management services if they are unstable medically or psychologically in order to ensure improvement in the child's complexity (Kathol 2010). The pediatric population poses unique challenges, in those children and youth, not of the age of consent, are completely dependent on others like family and caregivers in order to have their needs met (Matlow et al. 2006).

> Tips for Parents: It is important to bring to the attention of your care team all areas of challenge your child faces to help create the best plan of care, make sure to share the whole picture across your care providers as it could influence treatment decisions and collaborations.

> Tips for HealthCare Professionals: Specialists need to step back and consider how their component of the treatment plan might influence others, and/or how the child's environment relates to plan execution.

3.1.3 Care Coordination and Integrated Case Management

Poor care coordination is not a new or unique problem in healthcare and there are multiple efforts across areas of practice to improve. Care coordination should ensure collaboration and communication between the patient, family/caregiver and the healthcare team. When working with chronically ill and complex children, transition to the care of an adult parent or caregiver is an important facet in the process. Children with complex health conditions often are the victims of poor care coordination in both acute care and outpatient settings (Matlow et al. 2006). Often, no one is identified as a care coordinator, there are too many care coordinators, or those in place are poorly trained and incapable (Matlow et al. 2006).

Common opinion is that families and caregivers should take a leadership role in the care of the child, but often are ill-prepared due to health knowledge deficits (Matlow et al. 2006). As mentioned earlier, complex pediatric patients are often followed by multiple specialty providers and the primary pediatrician may also feel ill-equipped to play a pivotal role in the child's care coordination due to a lack of knowledge of certain medical conditions and communication with specialists is lacking (Matlow et al. 2006). Improved care coordination is essential to reduce serious consequences such as medication errors, duplication of services, and delay in services, morbidity and mortality.

Care coordination is improved by enhancing relationships: physician, specialists, ancillary providers, patients, families, and caregivers. Enhancing relationships also requires defining what works well for the patient and defining what limitations may be present (Matlow et al. 2006). Some organizations will form care coordination teams with each member assigned a particular area to address. This process seems to make sense as every member of the team has unique areas of strength and knowledge. This team concept can be successful if every member approaches communication and collaboration unilaterally. However, if this is not the method or approach, fragmented communication and coordination will continue.

3.1.4 Staffing

The authors of *The Integrated Case Management Training Manual: Assisting Complex Patients Regain Physical and Mental Health* advocate for one case manager working with a patient to assess, plan, and coordinate all care and services. The training itself provides a foundation for working with all health issues regardless of the clinician's background. One case manager addressing the needs of the patient is essential to the development of a relationship not only with the patient and family/caregiver, but also enhances the relationship with providers and will better define limitations present and what strategies will work best for the patient. One case manager can more effectively communicate and collaborate with all involved to remove barriers to improvement and ensure cohesive care coordination and transitions. The challenges of working with this population are discussed in this section as well as those of families and caregivers. The goal is to learn more about the need for improved care coordination and meeting the needs of families and caregivers.

3.1.5 Working with Children with Complex Health Issues

During the twentieth century, many effective therapies were developed to improve morbidity and mortality of life-threatening illnesses, infectious diseases, and congenital anomalies. Many children that suffered with these conditions did not survive to adolescence, but now often live to early adulthood and beyond (Lindsay and Grossman 2013). Chronic health conditions have biological, psychological, and social and health system implications for adults and children alike, but for children, developmental concerns are an equal implication. Historically, the approach taken to manage illness was organ system-based with emphasis on the physical disease; this does not address the non-biological aspects that are essential to attainment of optimal health.

Treatment of physical or biological conditions may result in cure, long-term improvement, or management of symptoms. Treatment for chronic conditions should be accompanied by preventative services, screenings, appropriate nutrition and physical activity. Often this involves the services of a case manager and/or care coordination team.

Tips for Parents: Ask the care provider team about training opportunities and about connection opportunities in the community.

Tips for HealthCare Professionals: Pediatric healthcare providers should, in collaboration with the family, prepare treatment strategies, monitor outcomes, coordinate visits with diagnostic tests, train caregivers, and educate other community service providers who will be involved with the child. Most important is to provide education and planning for emergencies to all involved in the child's care.

As part of the comprehensive care plan, assessments and monitoring for the potential of child abuse and neglect as children with disabilities are at greater risk. Integrated into the care plan and in general when working with families and caregivers, are acknowledgement of the family or caregiver's strengths, stressors that may be present, be ready to offer support and make referral for services that may provide parenting training, home health or respite care that may prevent any maltreatment of the child.

Children with special health care needs or complex conditions have very different experiences than those of healthy children. They are more likely to have altered development as a result of their condition. Developmental difficulties are more likely to occur during periods of normal transition like starting school or adolescence (Lindsay and Grossman 2013). An integrated case management assessment includes questions about a child's formal education as it is an important aspect of their life. Thanks to the laws under the Individuals with Disabilities Educational Act (IDEA), all children in the United States have access to early intervention and school age education suited to their needs and environment (Lindsay and Grossman 2013). More information about IDEA can be found at:

- www.ed.gov/offices/OSERS/IDEA/overview.html
- www.nichy.org/laws/idea.

Due to increasing demands on the public school system, some children may see delays or even prevention from receiving the services to which they are entitled. Healthcare professionals can step into advocate for these children to ensure they achieve their maximum educational potential.

Tips for Healthcare Professionals: the child's primary pediatrician can write on his/her prescription pad: "IDEA" then instruct parents/caregiver to take this to the child's school. This simple act can help facilitate and evaluation and implementation of educational services.

Psychological and/or behavioral problems may not be as common in children with complex health conditions but certainly are more prevalent than in their healthier peers. Psychological and/or behavioral problems are more likely to occur in adolescence (Matlow et al. 2006). Healthy adolescents will often behave differently due to their need to establish independence. In the child/adolescent with complex needs, their ability to achieve any level of independence may be hindered by their condition as they need assistance from parents/caregivers, teachers, and healthcare professionals. Children and adolescents with complex health needs should be routinely screened for psychological and behavioral problems with appropriate referral to mental health specialists.

Social issues and barriers can be the most debilitating to children with complex health needs, not to mention the impact on families and caregivers. Parents and caregivers find it difficult to balance their responsibilities: provide the needed care to the child with complex health needs, attend required healthcare appointments, be available during hospitalizations, giving time and attention to health siblings of the ill child, and maintain gainful employment. The economic health of family and caregivers is significantly affected by the needs of the child with complex health issues. The family and caregivers may have out of pocket expenses for office visits, hospitalizations, medications, therapies, and medical equipment which may prove to be a burden. This financial burden can be due to inadequate insurance coverage or simply the household income cannot support the expenses. Healthcare providers need to be cognizant of financial stressors.

Tips for Healthcare Professionals: routinely ask family and caregivers if they are having difficulties obtaining care and services.

Where appropriate, a referral to Medicaid or Children's Health Insurance Program should be made to see if the child with complex health needs would meet criteria for coverage by these agencies. Some children may be eligible for Supplemental Security Income. This program provides a monthly stipend and Medicaid coverage. In fact, there are certain conditions which make a child "presumably eligible" and benefits may be available during the formal evaluation period. Even if a child has private insurance as a result of one or more parent/caregiver's employment, do not assume the child will be ineligible. Children with private insurance coverage are often eligible for Medicaid as a secondary carrier. This secondary coverage can relieve some of the financial burden experienced as a result of co-pays, co-insurance or other non-covered services.

If Medicaid or other supplemental income is not an option, healthcare providers can guide families to explore managed care plans or medical homes. Managed care organizations focus on primary and preventative care, improved screening and risk assessment, comprehensive case management, and coordination with public health, education and social services. Managed Care organizations also implement gate-keeping arrangements to prevent over-utilization and duplication of services. A managed care plan can be a good option for families with limited financial resources.

Medical homes are an asset to integrated case management as the consistency of care provided in a setting familiar to all nuances of the child/family supports a holistic assessment and treatment plan for the individual. Medical homes are a system of care that seeks a shared responsibility with the patient, family, and community (Lindsay and Grossman 2013). Medical Homes provide accessible, comprehensive care which means preventative, primary and specialty services are available when needed, are well coordinated, family-centered, and culturally competent. This type of care system is especially beneficial to children with complex health needs and limited resources. Because all care and services are coordinated through the Medical Home, patients and families typically see a reduction in out-of-pocket expenses. All needed expertise is usually available; patients and families report improved satisfaction; and as the child grows, care transitions are also improved (Lindsay and Grossman 2013). The philosophy of the medical home is to focus on the child and his family rather than the illness. The care and services that children with special health needs require is much more time consuming than for the healthy child (Lindsay and Grossman 2013). This level of care can become less burdensome if providers allow for extended appointments; develop tracking systems that insure care coordination and continuity and the use of a problem-oriented medical record (Lindsay and Grossman 2013). Other members of the health care team, i.e. case managers, can assume the duties of care coordination so that the primary physician can focus on the child's special healthcare needs. The additional services provided by staff may be reimbursable with proper documentation and coding (Lindsay and Grossman 2013).

Tips for Parents: to learn more about Medical Homes for children visit The Center for Medical Home Implementation, http://www.medicalhomeinfo.org/.

As stated earlier, children with special health needs and chronic conditions are now more likely to grow into adulthood; in fact the estimated number is 90 % (Lindsay and Grossman 2013). Challenges arise in transitioning these children to self-sufficiency, financial independence and to adult healthcare providers.

Difficulties experienced as a result of this transition include (Lindsay and Grossman 2013):

- The healthcare environment in which they have been participating is geared toward school-aged children and not adolescence
- The adolescent transitioning to adulthood must cope with his or her emerging sexuality
- Children with special healthcare needs often have developmental challenges and are very dependent on their families and caregivers
- Because of dependence and possible developmental challenges, they may have difficulties making decisions about higher education or vocational pursuits.

3.1.6 Adolescent Transition and Integrated Case Management

Young adults transitioning to new healthcare providers may find it difficult to leave trusted, long-standing relationships to establish new provider relationships. The population of children and adolescents with special health needs is growing and our current healthcare system is not fully prepared to address these transitions (Lindsay and Grossman 2013). An approach of integrated case management is useful in the identification of issues and expectations of teens and families. Broaching the subject as early as is feasible, parents should be encouraged to begin thinking about their child's future as early as the toddler years (Lindsay and Grossman 2013).

Health care professionals should encourage parents to begin thinking about their child's future by asking questions like (Lindsay and Grossman 2013):

- "Have you thought about what Tommy might want to do after he finishes high school?"
- "Does Mary have any special interests or talents that you may want to explore as possible career choices?"

Healthcare providers can support and assist in the transition planning for adolescents by (Lindsay and Grossman 2013):

- Encouraging families and caregivers to allow children to try new and different activities
- Encouraging families and caregivers to enroll the child in programs that are typically for the child without challenges
- Contacting a vocational counselor for guidance before the adolescent seeks employment
- Encouraging families and caregivers, and the adolescent to think about possible part-time jobs, and/or volunteer work

- Helping families and caregivers understand the importance of the adolescent taking more responsibility with self-care, budgeting money, and participation in household chores
- Instructing families and caregivers to make sure the educational needs of the adolescent are included in the school's annual IEP to ensure appropriate transitions to the next educational level.

Transitions to adult healthcare providers should be focused on locating providers that will be committed to maximizing function and potential all through the life of the now adult with special health needs. Developmentally and behaviorally appropriate care and services should be of high quality due to the challenges of the transition (Lindsay and Grossman 2013).

3.1.7 Families and Caregivers

The case manager, utilizing an integrated approach to adolescents with special health needs, understands assessment and care plan actions are not limited to a child/adolescent's physical condition or even to only the child. Behavioral and developmental conditions and impairments contribute to overall complexity of the child or adolescent. These complex conditions affect the family dynamic as well. The cost of care for the complex child or adolescent can be a significant burden for families and caregivers. Families and caregivers also experience stressors related to the care demands of the child and the potential for less time spent with the rest of the family members. The needs of the families and caregivers are as important as those of the child. Being in a patient-centered healthcare environment will help ensure that the problems encountered by the child and family or caregivers are addressed and everyone is supported.

There is nothing more devastating for a parent than receiving the news that their child has been diagnosed with a chronic and potentially life-threatening illness. That devastation is increased when the child's physical illness is complicated by a developmental, behavioral and mental health disorder. Caring for a child with complex or special health needs is a long-term and life-altering event for parents and caregivers which results in multiple stressors that include emotional, psychological and financial consequences (McCabe and Scharf n.d.). These stressors occur at the time of diagnosis but continue and are often exacerbated as the child grows and develops, care needs change, and during acute illnesses and relapses (McCabe and Scharf n.d.). The parents and caregivers of the child with special health needs require a support system that can include family members and friends. A bigger challenge arises if a parent or caregiver lacks this type of support. Even in the presence of strong support, the family and caregiver can often feel isolated and alone when trying to cope with the multiple stressors related to their child's illness (McCabe and Scharf n.d.). Imagine if the parent or caregiver does not have a spouse, significant other, or other family members to assist.

Research shows that families with more stable relationships and adequate support have a higher quality of life but families with less stable relationships and less support will likely have a lower quality of life and experience increased conflict (McCabe and Scharf n.d.). Care coordination teams provide families and caregivers adequate support to addressing social, emotional and financial needs. If a parent or caregiver does not have the support of family and friends, healthcare providers can assist with finding other sources of support through the community, other parents and caregivers and the school systems. Families and caregivers may also benefit from family therapy for training in how to better cope, improve communication, and how to resolve conflict. Acquiring these skills and supports may also improve adherence to treatment (McCabe and Scharf n.d.).

Recommendations for families and caregivers to improve needed support: (McCabe and Scharf n.d.):

- Ask healthcare providers if volunteers are available to provide training, education and support, especially during the early stages of diagnosis
- Make sure the healthcare provider demonstrates empathy and understanding
- Don't hesitate or be afraid to tell the healthcare provider that help is needed
- Inform teachers, counselors, and the school principal of the child's illness, healthcare needs and the need for help and support
- Ask healthcare providers if support groups are available that include others who are going through similar situations.

One of the most common challenges for families and caregivers is managing the care of their child (Leis-Newman 2011). The often overwhelming responsibilities of the child's care interfere with the ability to cope, resulting in depression. If a child's primary caregiver is depressed, treatment adherence for the child is decreased (Leis-Newman 2011). Anxiety and depression in parents and caregivers results directly from the stressors related to the child's care and limited support, even if the parent or caregiver has a spouse (Leis-Newman 2011). Parents and caregivers experiencing anxiety and depression should access care for themselves (Leis-Newman 2011). Improved adherence to treatment and overall health in children with special health needs was seen when parents and caregivers got treatment for their own anxiety and depression according to an international study done on children with CF and their parents (Leis-Newman 2011).

3.1.8 Taking Care of Caregivers

Family and caregivers of children with special health needs do not always have large supportive families, a circle of friends willing to help, or adequate financial resources. But every parent or caregiver devotes all to care for their child, but the burden can be overwhelming, not to mention the additional responsibility for spouses, other children, elderly parents, and work outside the home. Eventually, even the strongest of parents or caregivers will feel emotionally, physically, and

mentally drained. Parent/caregiver self-care is essential in order to continue to care
for the child. The following are some simple suggestions that might families and
caregivers better cope with this long-term commitment (KidsHealth n.d.):

- *Find at least an hour or two each week to be alone*—away from the child and
  other responsibilities: take a nap, read, take a walk, have lunch or dinner with a
  friend, go shopping… whatever will help achieve relaxation.
- *Eat well*—avoid fast food if possible. Keep healthy snacks on hand especially if
  significant time is spent in clinics or hospitals. Let friends bring homemade
  food to the hospital or home.
- *Get regular exercise*—walking, riding a bike and yoga are good activities and
  easy ways to get exercise. Exercise releases chemicals in the brain called
  endorphins. Endorphins give one a feeling of well-being and can help relieve
  anxiety and prevent depression.
- *Try to stay organized*—keep all information about the child's health in one place:
  schedules of appointments, provider names and phone numbers, and insurance
  information. Keep a notebook to track things about the child's condition that are
  of concern and may need to be discussed with healthcare providers.
- *Don't be afraid to ask for help*—let those that offer to bring dinner, do shopping, other errands, or spend time with the child's other siblings. Most people
  that offer help are sincere in their offers and by allowing them to help, they will
  feel as though they are making a meaningful contribution.
- *Find a support group*—talk to a social worker at the clinic or hospital and ask
  that they can help find a group with participants that have similar experiences.
  Feelings of isolation are eliminated when experiences are shared.

Tips for Parents: If as a parent or caregiver is having difficulty managing all the responsibilities, and efforts to relieve stress have been unsuccessful, seek professional help.

In order to prevent disabling anxiety or depression, the care coordination team
may recommend family or individual counseling to help process feelings and find
family strategies to cope.

How to recognize the signs of anxiety or depression (KidsHealth n.d.):

- Changes in sleep or appetite: eating too much or too little; sleeping too much or
  too little
- Avoiding seeing friends or other social activities
- Increased feelings of anxiousness, nervousness, difficulty concentrating
- Crying often
- Increased irritability: feeling angry, irritated, lack of patience
- Feeling lost, alone, empty.

The role of the care coordination team is supporting identification and
acknowledgement of feelings of stress and developing a plan with the family. The
case manager can help to identify resources, providing support and encouragement
to the family centered plan. Families need attention as well as the child with
special healthcare needs.

3.1.9 Summary

Children and adolescents with complex health needs require medical, psychological, developmental, and social care and services. Barriers in any one of these areas leads to an increase in complexity and poor health outcomes. Healthcare professionals working with this population must be cognizant of the interconnectivity of these domains and make sure that all are addressed based on priority, but with the understanding that none should be ignored. One primary care manager to address all issues, with the needed resources as hand, would be preferred to ensure appropriate care coordination, transition, support, and maintenance of the relationship between patient and family or caregiver.

Parents and caregivers experience high levels of stress that can lead to impaired physical and psychological health. Providing parents and caregivers appropriate assistance and support ensures their stable health and ultimately improved or stabilized health for their child. The needs of parents and caregivers are as important as that of the child: again recognize the interconnectivity of physical, psychological and social issues. Healthcare professionals need to provide care, support and resources to families; families and caregivers need to ask for help and know where and how to access needed resources.

References

Chen, A. Y., Schrager, S. M., & Mangione-Smith, R. (2012, February 13). Quality measures for primary care of complex pediatric patients. *Pediatrics, 129*(3). Retrieved October, 2013, from http://pediatrics.aappublications.org/content/early/2012/02/08/peds.2011-0026.

Kathol, R. P. (2010). *The integrated case managment manual: Assisting complex patients regaine physical and mental health.* New York: Springer Publishing.

KidsHealth. (n.d.). *Taking Care of You: Support for Caregivers.* Retrieved July 1, 2014, from KidsHealth: www.kidshealth.org/parents/system/ill/caregivers.tml?tracking=P_RelatedArticle.

Leis-Newman, E. (2011, March). *Caring for Chronically Ill Children.* Retrieved July 1, 2014, from American Psychological Association: www.apa.org/monitor/2011/03/ill-children.aspx.

Lindsay, K., & Grossman, M. (2013, August 23). *Children with Special Health Care Needs.* Retrieved January 2, 2014, from UpToDate: www.uptodate.com/children-with-special-health-care-needs?topicKey=PEDS%2F2840&elapsedTimeMs=5&source=seelink&view.

Matlow, A., Wright, J., Zimmerman, B., Thompson, K., & Valente, M. (2006, April). How can the principles of complexity science be applied to improve the coordination of care for complex pediatric patients? *Quality and SAfety in Healthcare, 15*(2), 85–88. Retrieved October 31, 2013, from www.ncbi.nlm.nih.gov/pmc/articles/PMC2464825/.

McCabe, P., PhD., & Scharf, C. (n.d.). *Buliding Stronger, Healthier Families When a Child is Chronically Ill: A Guide for School Personnel.* Retrieved July 1, 2014, from NASP: www.nasponline.org/publications/cq/36/1/families.aspx.

Chapter 4
Legislative and Policy Movement

4.1 Policy and Action

Policy and action advocating for children's health issues comes in many forms.

- Advocacy groups representing certain diagnosis
- Advocacy groups for certain vulnerable populations based on evidence of health disparities
- Legislation supporting specific rights and benefit provisions
- Professional organizations oversight indicating how groups must govern, document and deliver care.

All these groups impact the ultimate delivery of care to children in our country.

Care coordination has emerged as one of the most important aspects in the care of children with special heath care needs yet when physicians are polled they indicate lack of staff and community/government agency services as a common reason for not providing care coordination services (Gupta et al. 2004). Advocacy and policy to support workforce and program development will be necessary as policy inclusion to enable widespread care coordination adoption across pediatric practices.

As a parent or healthcare professional, the important message is understanding how the family situation can be the impetus for change, so it is important to speak out. The follow-up point is that there is advantage in promoting your cause/issue with groups of like-minded people. In grassroots efforts to impact policy, whether at your school system, state or the national government level, involving people to contact those in power over the issue (school board, state or federal legislators) do influence action. Since others have mastered the art of lobbying and media contact, it is best to use connections with family and professional advocacy groups to support your cause in addition to your own family and local contacts. This chapter will briefly introduce existing national and state legislation impacting coordination of care for children in the U.S. as well as pointing to connections for advocacy groups.

© The Author(s) 2015   39
J. Treadwell et al., *Case Management and Care Coordination*,
SpringerBriefs in Child Health, DOI 10.1007/978-3-319-07224-1_4

A prime example comes from the work occurring through the Assuring Better Child Health and Development (ABCD) Program. The Commonwealth Fund has funded ABCD programs across states to positively impact delivery of early child development services for low-income children and their families by strengthening primary health care services and systems support. The experience with implementation illustrated that policy improvements were more successful when they were integral to the initiative and were part of the initial start of a project. The other barometer of success is support from senior state government leaders (Kaye and May 2013).

4.2 National Policy

At the national level, policy most recently impacting care coordination is the Patient Protection Affordable Care Act (www.HealthCare.gov/laresources/index.html). The Affordable Care Act (ACA) impacts children and youth through removal of lifetime financial limits, the facilitation of 2.5 million young adults in maintaining access to coverage (by being able to stay on their parents insurance plan), and the emphasis of care coordination within the language of the bill specific to models of care, care transitions, and access to needed services. The ACA also contained provisions for the Centers for Medicaid and Medicare Strategies (CMS) to implement an Innovation Center, supporting research into new health care models that strengthen quality and support innovative strategies to address chronic disease and vulnerable populations. The key goal of the Affordable Care Act is improved population management using value-based strategies inclusive of care coordination (Llewellyn 2013). One item missing in the ACA, relevant to care coordination is the definition of the qualifications of the people providing the coordination services. To protect the public from inexperienced or uninformed people engaging in care coordination activity at the potential financial and safety risk of children, clarification is necessary.

There are many important pieces of national legislation that impact coordination of health care for children. The Health Insurance Portability and Accountability Act (HIPAA) removes the preexisting condition requirement from health coverage and protects the privacy of health information by requiring security measures of people and entities that maintain health information. This includes anyone conducting care coordination activity. Healthcare information can however and should be exchanged between healthcare providers associated with a child's care coordination. Specifically, the George Washington University School of Public Health and Health Services (SPHHS) has researched the exchange of healthcare information as it relates to potential barriers or assists of health information laws and health system improvements for children and adolescents under Medicaid's Early and Periodic Screening, Diagnosis and Treatment (EPSDT) benefit. What they found was that information on treatments and screening is supported without additional consent across providers to aid in seamless care for children (Perna 2013).

There are five main pieces of federal legislation addressing both education and health of children requiring care coordination beyond the legislative provisions for health coverage specified under Medicaid and State Children's Health Insurance (CHIP) Programs and the associated State Waiver programs. Some of the Waiver programs require efforts of care coordination, however all Medicaid and CHIP recipients can ask for, and receive, case management services. Acknowledging that education and health are intertwined in the total well-being of the child, the Individuals with Disabilities Education Act (IDEA), No Child Left Behind Act (NCLB), Section 504 of the Rehabilitation Act, American Disabilities Act (ADA) and Assistive Technology Act (ATA) seek to define and protect rights of a child to receive education and health.

The Individuals with Disabilities Education Act (IDEA) provides school districts federal monies to support education of children with disabilities. The law specifies parental rights and requires states provide free public education in the least restrictive setting for the child. The No Child Left Behind Act (NCLB) focuses on the accountability of special education programs to ensure oversight and coordination for students with disabilities (Yell et al. 2005, p. 34). Supporting these education programs are state oversight entities which are accountable back to the Office of Special Education Programs (OSEP), which will direct healthcare professionals to each states' available programming. These programs include Parent Training and Information Centers (PTI) in every state to supports projects providing information and technical assistance to families of children with disabilities.

Under Section 504 of the Rehabilitation Act, school districts are required to provide a free appropriate public education (FAPE) to qualified students who have a physical or mental impairment that limits life activities. This means special education and related educational aids assist in language and communication. Similarly the Americans with Disabilities Act (ADA) requires daycare and schools have to make reasonable modifications to integrate children with disabilities into their programs unless doing so would require a fundamental alteration of their program. Both of those laws are supported by the Assistive Technology Act (ATA) which enables the provision of devices including wheelchairs, communication devices, durable medical equipment, lifts, accessibility adaptations for both home and school, and equipment to help in recreation and study (e.g. magnifiers, reachers, large keyboards).

Case managers and the care coordination team will reference these policy and specific legislation as necessary when developing a child's plan of care. Familiarity with policy helps support the developmental needs of a child in areas of both health and education. Since over one in three children were covered through a federal benefit program in 2012, the public health insurance benefit provisions are an important component of coordinating children's health services (Sebelius 2013). Nuances to coverage and qualifications vary from state to state. These benefit provisions are important as they serve as the components to be coordinated for the child's plan of care. Children with commercial health coverage have like program provisions which can be referenced through the insurance carrier.

Tips for Parents: If your child needs assistance with school access or activities, schedule a meeting to explain the needed assistive equipment or adaption asking for an explicit timeframe for action. Document the meeting date and attendees.

Tips for HealthCare Professionals: Providers can be of assistance to families by providing letters of explanation for adaptive requests to ensure continuity of care and support of any disability when the child is in the classroom.

Another national influence on care coordination involves professional certification and how our country defines who calls themselves a care coordinator or case manager. Certification is presently available to qualified professionals seeking to evidence their experience and understanding of case management and care coordination. The Accredited Care Management Association adopted a position statement proclaiming that by the year 2016, nurses and social workers should attain status not only through their professional license but also through case management certification however, there is no requirement at the present time for certification of a person uses the title of case manager of care coordinator. An example of entities providing education and examination for certification include: the Case Management Society of America, American Case Management Association, the American Association of Managed Care Nurses, the American Nurses Credentialing Center Nursing Case Management credential, and the American Academy of Case Management. Individuals who perform non-professional care coordination services as part of a team should be able to demonstrate training through certificate completion of a Community Health Worker program or from Patient Advocate training, indicating education and understanding of family-centered care coordination. For reasons of child safety and efficacy, it is an issue presented now to legislators in state and federal venues requesting clear definitions for individuals performing care coordination.

Tips for Parents: Ask the case manager performing assessments and care planning for your child, about their educational and certification status. Verify credentials to ensure you are receiving support from a qualified professional.

Tips for Health Care Professionals: When selecting partners for conducting care coordination, or when hiring a care coordinator, look for certification status as well as a non-restricted professional license to protect your patients.

4.3 State Policy

Beyond the issue of health insurance coverage, differences exist at the state level in regards to special programming and resources. State waivers offering richer benefit packages are available in some states. Specific information on care in specific states can be found through the National Academy for State Health. The national strategy includes improved screening which results in more children identified with needs for coordination across the continuum of health services. Individualized care planning and cross systems planning is promoted within the state Health and Human Services Commissions to utilize all resources and be as child/family centered as possible for maximum results. State policy is supporting information and technology infrastructure that will facilitate improved coordination long term. Those strategies will be essential in times of natural disaster when coordination needs to extend beyond a local community and perhaps even state. States have acknowledged addressing the health and developmental needs of children and families requires linkage across communities and monitoring of those referrals just as satisfaction and cost outcomes are measured. States are engaging their managed care organization partners to provide evidence of those outcomes.

Payment for Care Coordination services is a changing area although the Centers for Medicaid and Medicare Services did approve in 2013 for 2014, reimbursement supporting care management "outside the routine office interaction to promote high quality care and efficiency" in Medicare for physicians and non-physicians. State adoption into Medicaid will be an issue to follow across states.

Another potential state issue impacting care coordination is that of multistate licensure. Case Managers are healthcare professionals licensed within a state. Nurses and social workers are regulated on a state-by state basis. This means that a case manager must hold a license in a state where the patient lives. It is common for individuals living near state borders to receive care in that bordering state. For case managers attempting to coordinate care, this can place their license at risk. Acquiring a license in each state is administratively and financially burdensome. Twenty-four states, per the Multi-State Licensure National Council of State Boards of Nursing have agreed to enter into a compact, recognizing nursing licensure across states. Adoption by states who have not yet accepted is necessary to protect case managers. There is a belief that interest in the advancement of telemedicine (which transcends state lines) and physician action to move their licensing to multi-state status will add strength to this issue, compelling adoption in additional states over the next few years. The goal for states is an integrated care coordination infrastructure to deliver optimal pediatric health care. As described by Antonelli, McAllister, and Popp, in their framework for high performing pediatric care coordination, this will require attention to all levels within the health care system and across multiple sectors of the community (2009). In addition to outcomes measures, states and local communities must develop program and workforce infrastructure, education, policy support, and financing (Antonelli et al. 2009).

4.4 Advocacy

There is a difference between gaps in coordination of services and a lack of programming or coverage for a service. The care coordination team, in concert with the family and health professionals should be able to address communication and coordination in care and services between insurance coverage, waiver offerings, and community services. When holes in coverage or benefits exist that impair continuity of care or adequate healthcare provision, advocacy groups become essential in initiating changes to existing policy or working on new policy creation.

This requires a strong voice, for example an advocacy organization. Family Voices, is a national organization, respected in children's healthcare policy that helps families make informed decisions. As a trusted resource, Family Voices advocates for improved public policy and builds partnerships across organizations, providers and families. The family and care coordination team will find Family Voices a dependable resource for advocacy and support.

Another vital role of the advocacy groups is the voice of experience that comes from parents who have raised children with the same or similar diagnoses or circumstances. Sharing how the accommodation of life plays out in one family can be immensely important to families trying to cope with the needs of one child with special healthcare needs, and balancing needs of other children and family members. Tips on arranging furniture and supply storage can help families improve their day just as training on advocacy, information on waiver program availability and methods to integrate adolescents into an adult provider system. Parent to Parent is an organization that can make those important connections between families. State chapters of the national Parent to Parent organization identify a match of experienced support parents that can help with both needed information and emotional support. They provide additional networking opportunities and educational offerings as well as a committed resource for families with children who have a special health care need, disability, or mental health issue. Other great resources can be found through the websites of the National Center for Medical Home Implementation and The Maternal and Child Health Library at Georgetown University. The Medical Home site has resources for parents and practitioners surrounding how to be develop effective care plans, shared decisions on contact plans and effective strategies of family inclusion. The Georgetown University site hosts disease specific information for parents as well as professional and school resources, all focused on providing coordinated support for family-centered care.

No section on advocacy would be complete without information on social media and grassroots efforts. To be effective in our communities, advocating for our children, we need to identify and support good policies and move into action opposing those that are not. Grassroots efforts are about pulling together the mobilization of friends and families who care about children's health at a specific time. Writing a letter or email or calling to a state or federal legislator, attending a rally, testifying before a committee, and informing friends and local organizations so they can speak up as well. Legislators can understand and relate when they can hear a real story about how policy affects children's health and family life. Similarly, the media can carry stories to inform people who would be willing to help in grassroots efforts due to their aligned beliefs about children. The entire care coordination team has an opportunity to work with the media in telling the story of how coordination decreases fragmentation, improves clinical and financial outcomes of care and increases family satisfaction.

References

Antonelli, R., McAllister, J., & Popp, J. (2009). *Making Care Coordination a Critical Component of the Pediatric Health System: A Multidisciplinary Framework.* The Commonwealth Fund. Retrieved from http://www.commonwealthfund.org/Publications/Fund-Reports/2009/May/Making-Care-Coordination-a-Critical-Component-of-the-Pediatric-Health-System. aspx#citation.

Gupta, V., O'Connor, K., & Quezada-Gomez, C. (2004, May). Care coordination services in pediatric practices. *Pediatrics, 113*(4), 1517–1521. Retrieved from http://pediatrics.aappublications.org/content/113/Supplement_4/1517.full.

Llewellyn, A. (2013, October). Case management playing a key role in the advancement of clinical integration. *Case in Point,* Retrieved July 1, 2014 from http://www.dorlandhealth.com/dorland-health-articles/Case-Management-Playing-a-Key-Role-in-the-Advancement-of-Clinical-Integration

Kaye, N., & May, J. (2013). State Policy Improvements that Support Effective Identification of Children At-Risk for Developmental Delay: Findings from the ABCD Screening Academy, National Academy for State Health Policy. Retrieved from http://www.nashp.org/improving-policy#sthash.Tulplmqj.dpuf.

Perna, G. (2013, September). Researchers Explore Pediatric Care Coordination with Health Information Regulations.

Sebelius, K. (2013). The Department of Health and Human Services 2013 Annual Report on the Quality of Care for Children in Medicaid and CHIP. Retrieved from http://www.medicaid.gov/Medicaid-CHIP-Program-Information/By-Topics/Quality-of-Care/Downloads/2013-Ann-Sec-Rept.pdf.

The Social Work Leadership Institute of the New York Academy of Medicin. (2009, August). *Who is Qualified to Coordinate Care?* A report prepared for the New York State Department of Health and The State Office for the Aging. New York, NY. Retrieved from http://socialworkleadership.org/nsw/index.php.

Yell, M. L., Drasgow, E., & Lowrey, K. A. (2005). No child left behind and students with autism spectrum disorders. *Focus on Autism and Other Developmental Disabilities, 20*(3), 130–139.

Part II
Implications for Policy and Practice
(Emerging Science and Best Practices—
Practical Application)

Chapter 5
Children with Special Health Care Needs and Their Families Achieving Shared Care-Planning and Coordination of Care

5.1 Introduction

The Patient and Family-Centered Medical Home grounds US Maternal and Child Health Bureau policy and represents a strategic priority of the American Academy of Pediatrics (AAP) as noted in their 2008 American Academy of Pediatrics Medical Home Initiatives for Children With Special Needs Project Advisory Committee (AAP 2008; Strickland et al. 2004). As a model of care the pediatric medical home gained strong momentum during the last decade of the twentieth Century; it is considered the standard of primary care for all children including children and youth with special health care needs (CYSHCN). CYSHCN are those who have or are at risk for chronic physical, developmental, behavioral, or emotional conditions that require health and related services of a type or an amount beyond that required by children generally (McPherson et al. 1998). Today the AAP states that all children deserve a medical home—providing accessible, continuous, comprehensive, family-centered, coordinated, compassionate, and culturally effective care (National Center for Medical Home Implementation 2014).

Many refer to the implementation of medical home standards in today's clinical care settings as "transformation". That is, a makeover from what capabilities exists to those described by the medical home model that should be present and experienced by all patients. In pediatrics, patient and family centered care is the term more frequently used to show the importance to child health when the entire family is considered. In pediatric primary care, differentiation is often made between medical home transformation focused on CYSHCN, and improvements, which focus on all children. This difference is often communicated in a manner suggesting that the meaning when they say "all children" does not include children with special health care needs. The medical home is a standard of quality care for *all* children; children and youth who live with chronic health conditions make up about 18 % of *all* children. Therefore, the medical home and all efforts to

© The Author(s) 2015
J. Treadwell et al., *Case Management and Care Coordination*,
SpringerBriefs in Child Health, DOI 10.1007/978-3-319-07224-1_5

transform primary care and achieve the goals of the Triple Aim (better care, population health, and costs per capita) should be all inclusive (Berwick et al. 2008).

Studies of medical home transformation refer to innovations that are currently being tested in practice in real time, or improvements that are needed but have not been fully tested by the rigor of everyday primary care practice. Examples of such medical home innovations include open access, staff huddles, group visits, co-management agreements, patient portals, and more. Care coordination is a most consistently highlighted as an important and needed innovation. Historically consensus on the definition of care coordination has been elusive. Care coordination, case management and care management are terms, which are often used interchangeably. Subsequently these terms have become the subject of discussions and differentiation with papers aiming for or seeking clarity of meaning among the many nuanced references.

The meaning of care coordination, and of case or care management, continues to evolve and change. This may be the result of care coordination implementation in the medical home with identification of what works best. It may also occur as a result of program leaders shaping it to meet expectations or intentions of an improvement or reform initiative. This chapter will focus on care coordination, with an intention to emphasize patient and family partnership and engagement, rather than management of "care" or of "cases". Families have frequently been quoted as stating that they are not "cases" and that they do not want to be "managed". Family advocates encourage professionals to acknowledge and respect parents and caregivers in their efforts to coordinate a child's care in the context of what it takes to raise and nurture them. Family-centered care coordination takes an approach of looking to and asking the patient and family for cues about what coordination they want or will take the lead on and which areas that they will need help. Care coordination can be described as a set of functions; these functions are then to be negotiated and shared among the family and team.

Care coordination has been described as glue, or the element that holds people, processes and tools together leading to better care. But family-centered care coordination is far more actionable than glue; its core competencies and key coordinating functions generate real activities to help the varied people and processes in different parts of the system to collaborate and integrate effectively. The metaphor of oil and gears is more apt as care coordination applies the emollient to effectively move care forward continuously meeting identified goals and plans.

5.2 Background

Foundational building blocks for high quality care coordination in the medical home can be found among a select articles and policy briefs of the last decade. The work of this literature offers an idealized framework from which to develop and provide care coordination with infants, children, youth and families. The AAP lays down these building blocks with two key policy statements, one on the medical home and the second on care coordination (AAP 2004; AAP Commitee on Children with Disabilities 2005) Cooley and McAllister bring these policy statements to life with their application and description of the model for improvement in the pediatric primary care medical home (Cooley and McAllister 2004). Antonelli and colleagues add their care coordination time study including an analysis of care coordination activities across a team, functions and methods, and whether payment could be linked to the named core activities of practice based care coordination (Antonelli et al. 2008). Stille and Antonelli (2004) added to these further descriptions of care coordination and co-management among families, primary care clinicians and specialists. Looman and colleagues (2013) link the need for coordination to the existing skill sets of advanced practice registered nurses who are filling current and pressing workplace needs. Antonelli et al. 2009 merged their interests and perspectives to put forth a pediatric framework for care coordination which includes a definition described below, outlines competencies, and lists critical care coordination functions (See Table 5.1).

Care coordination is an essential element of the family-centered medical home model. By definition pediatric care coordination is a patient and family-centered, assessment-driven, team-based activity designed to meet the needs of children and youth while enhancing the caregiving capabilities of families (Antonelli et al. 2009). Care coordination addresses interrelated medical, social, developmental, behavioral, educational, environmental and financial needs to achieve optimal health and wellness outcomes.

5.3 Care Coordination: A Medical Home Transformation Essential Element

Medical home transformation was the topic of a 2010 Agency for Healthcare Research and Quality call for proposals. The context at the time was one of the initiations of numerous adult primary care medical home projects in the wake of Transformed, a national medical home demonstration effort (Nutting et al. 2009). The study "Transformation in the Pediatric Medical Home: What Drives Change" was one of fourteen projects funded to collect and analyze practice characteristics contributing to "accomplished transformation" (McAllister et al. 2013). The notion that transformation is ever complete was a difficult concept to absorb by the twelve pediatric practices studied. Working on medical home improvements for 7 years these primary care teams were still busy improving. In fact, when interviewed each practice related ideas more fitting with continuous improvement than completed transformation. Four essential elements of effective medical home change are described in this study and include (1) quality improvement, (2) family centered care, (3) teamwork and (4) care coordination. These highly functioning

Table 5.1 Essential care
coordination functions

Family-centered care coordination:
1. Provides separate visits and care coordination interactions
2. Manages continuous communications
3. Completes/analyzes assessments
4. Develops care plans with families
5. Manages/tracks tests, referrals, and outcomes
6. Coaches patients/families
7. Integrates critical care information
8. Supports/facilitates care transitions
9. Facilitates team meetings
10. Uses health information technology

practices enjoy a significant degree of senior leadership with encouragement and support for their medical home efforts. Their quality improvement initiatives benefit from devoted time and dedication to their tasks. Families of children with special health care needs serve as their improvement partners. Lead clinicians, care coordinators and families report frequent new discoveries about how to best design and deliver team-based care. While no team employed a designated coordinator of care at the beginning of their improvement efforts, today all but one of twelve practices employs one or more devoted care coordinators (McAllister et al. 2013).

There are numerous care coordination lessons to be learned from this study. Using a methodology of coded qualitative interviews, of over almost 6,000 coded quotes, over 4,000 are linked to coordination of care. Care coordination is best achieved in the context of relationships. The four essential elements are interdependent. Quality improvement takes a team. Teamwork must be valued with its work appreciated as vital. This necessitates highly effective team habits such as frequent meetings, agenda setting, adequate time for effective communication and accountable follow up of assigned tasks. More often than not the lead clinician serves as team leader, but decisions are rarely made without family members and care coordinators input and agreement (McAllister et al. 2013).

The relationship among the child, family and primary care clinician is key to a successful medical home. The contract of this relationship is that patients and families are empowered and supported to manage and coordinate care in partnership with their primary care team. Fundamental to family-centered care and to effective quality improvement is direct feedback from families to inform team-based care including care coordination. The child and family perspective; their current experience of care; and ideas they have for what would make care better are questions which need to be asked on a regular basis? The transformation study referenced revealed numerous developed family-friendly care processes and materials of which their use became care coordination roles and functions. The teams also tested new and specific approaches to care coordination including pre-visit contacts, separate care coordination visits and access options, and jointly created plans of care to name a few. The clinicians, families, and coordinators would debrief as a group, adapt approaches, re-plan for another try and/or mark any successful outcomes accordingly (McAllister et al. 2013).

Strong teamwork is a product of quality improvement, family engagement and care coordination. Among these four essential elements, you truly cannot have one with out the other (Fig. 5.1). Another medical home effort, the National Safety Net Medical Home Initiative reports similar findings (2014).

5.4 Putting It All Together for Care Coordination Implementation

Shared plans of care have gained wide attention as a method very needed and when well executed instrumental to integrate multiple people, sources of information and input, and all recommended next steps with clear accountabilities. Plans of care are being looked to as a key tool to help coalesce multiple inputs into a comprehensive approach with clearly laid out steps and easy to use. The Center for Medical Home Improvement (1997–2013) collected and published work related to medical home improvements (Antonelli et al. 2009)

CMHI organized data collected from families as follows: we would like a system of care that provides us with:

(1) Efficient access to the practice with an identified personal contact
(2) A team who knows our family history and preferences well, and
(3) Continuous care coordination using a jointly created, and effectively implemented, plan of care.

It is clear that families would like a distilled summary of their child's diagnosis and treatments, and a plan of care to effectively frame—who their child is, and what their strengths are. Families also want their pivotal role as the true constant and expert in the life and care of their child to be highlighted. Clinicians have also voiced their opinions, asking for a swift, comprehensive and accurate snapshot, or medical summary, to assist them in the delivery of care delivered under real time pressures and constraints. Shared plans of care are on deck as the next medical home "innovation" to develop and test. Will existing care coordination help us to achieve these aspirations or will these developments lead to better care coordination, or both?

In 2012 The Lucille Packard Foundation for Children's Health (LPFCH) funded first the Center for Medical Home Improvement and subsequently the Indiana University's School of Medicine, Children's Health Services Research Division to work towards a consensus process for planned coordinated care, using plans of care. The charge was to define and describe the critical dimensions of a comprehensive integrated plan of care. The result is a LPFCH Brief; the brief outlines a model for coordination of care using plans of care. It includes underlying consensus principles (Table 5.2), a step-by-step approach to shared care-planning, and

Fig. 5.1 Four essential
elements of pediatric medical
home transformation

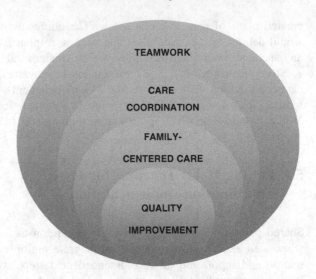

a companion learning guide for teams to use as they uptake the steps of the model (McAllister et al. 2014). The plan of care is conceptualized as a blend of traditional "medical summary" data merged with a "negotiated actions" component to capture goals, strategies, actions, person responsible and related accountabilities.

The ten underlying principles about health system capacity, family-centered partnerships, and practice context set the stage for effective comprehensive and integrated care planning. These are reiterated in Table 5.2.

When these 10 core assumptions are fully implemented, the benefits of having and using a shared plan of care will be realized and they are predicted to promote the following positive results:

- Youth and families who are empowered to self-advocate and partner with providers/professionals as full team members
- Close alignment of patient and family goals with critical medical advice towards better clinical outcomes
- Efforts of all youth, family, providers, specialists, community partners, and other care givers including emergency providers are integrated around commonly shared goals
- Care planning results from important youth/family engagement; as partners families and professionals create and implement the plan of care together
- Access to care and information is facilitated for ease and clarity
- Safer care is a result of improved continuity and accuracy, consistent emergency responses and clarification of actions (already) tried and those not yet tried
- A framework and discipline is then established for professionals which directs their coordinating interactions and addresses standards set by quality recognizing organizations

Table 5.2 Shared plan of care principles adapted from "McAllister et al. (2014)

Better care, population health and cost effective benefits will be realized when:
1. Children, youth and families are actively engaged in their care
2. Communication with and among their medical home team is clear, frequent and timely
3. Providers/team members base their patient and family assessments on a full understanding of child, youth and family needs, strengths, history, and preferences
4. Youth, families, health care providers, and their community partners have strong relationships characterized by mutual trust and respect
5. Family-centered care teams can access the information they need to make shared, informed decisions
6. Family-centered care teams use a Shared Plan of Care, which includes shared goals with negotiated actions; all partners understand the Sharing Care-Planning process, their individual responsibilities and related accountabilities
7. The team monitors progress against goals, provides feedback and adjusts the plan of care on an on-going basis to ensure that the plan is well implemented
8. Team members anticipate, prepare and plan for all transitions (e.g. early intervention to school; hospital to home; pediatric to adult care)
9. The Shared Care Plan is systematized as a common document; it is used consistently by every provider within an organization, and by all providers across organizations
10. Care is subsequently well coordinated across all involved organizations/systems

- A model and plan of care process guides all care coordination activities with built-in tracking and monitoring to show progress against goals and plans (McAllister 2014).

5.5 Challenges

Time, payment and conflicting political pressures continue to challenge medical home transformation; related studies show us that those who daily deliver care can overcome some, but not all of these challenges. The success of achieving a jointly created and effectively shared plan of care is impacted by these challenges. Technology is another looming challenge but it is also a great opportunity. While technology is responsible for bringing information to the fingertips of end users in unprecedented ways, the electronic systems used in many health networks are still not facile enough to enable real-time planned, coordinated care with the development and use of medical summaries and negotiated next steps. Teams invest significant time to develop a plan of care, yet their efforts are not fully supported by technological tools. They need help with auto-updating, tracking and monitoring functions and families want the "product" created from these electronic systems to be accessible and succinct. They in turn use such a plan of care in their informed interactions with other providers. Technology falls short in putting current and accurate information in front of the team, into the hands of the family, and out to community partners and specialists in real time. Accessible, searchable, and retrievable care coordination data and plans of care is a reachable goal and this challenge can and should be addressed with urgency.

New, under the Affordable Care Act, and as a standard of meaningful use certification, is the mandate to incorporate the components of care planning into the "Continuity of Care Document" (CCD). This standard applies to both ambulatory and inpatient care. A high quality plan of care or "care record" should take the form of a shared plan of care, be developed in partnership with patients and families, be jointly implemented and have accountabilities documented. Families clearly need and want the guidance to be found in the plan of care, yet this is still not easy to deliver efficiently. Technologies that support the team to develop, continuously update, and share plans of care with families and their identified community partners remains elusive.

5.6 Tips for Teams to Think About

There are many resources with tips that support families and practice teams to work together (ref see IPFCC, medical home info, PCPCC, etc.). The following tips speak to the collaborative practice of medical home improvement teams:

(1) Ask and answer questions. There is a saying that "one does not have because one does not ask". Asking is more often, than not, a good idea. If you are unsure, ask yourself what is the worst that could happen? The answer may give you confidence to proceed. The assumption is that care coordination is best delivered as a team-based service; to be a team members (families, clinicians, coordinators and others) need to form relationships. Relationships involve getting to know one another, which require a willingness to ask, and answer questions about what is important to children, young adults, and families or what the clinical team members need to know or understand to perform their roles well. Care coordination is assessment driven, being assessment *driven* means using a process to look at strengths and gaps. Asking is being informed and being informed leads to better understanding of one another's perspectives.

- For the clinical care team this means asking what is needed, what is missing, what strengths are at the ready to help achieve goals.
- For families you may want to know:
  - Examples of how the practice partners and learns from families in an ongoing manner
  - Is there a no non-clinician staff person to be your practice contact
  - Is there a care team who can help you with coordination of care
  - Will the team partner with you to develop a plan of care for your child?
  - Will they help you to communicate with other pertinent partners (school staff or specialists)

(2) Select care coordination individuals for their attitude as well as their skill set. Identify and address your team/care coordination goals. Who make the best care coordinators? Many health system leaders ask this question about what professional disciplines are best prepared to be excellent care coordinators.

- Hire for attitude, family centered beliefs, and care coordination functional skills; this is the answer with the most traction. Some groups have found that nurses make wonderful care coordinators, others use social workers, and still others have the opportunity to draw from both. Families are also serving in related coordinating roles. Different individuals may carry out separate functions of care coordination but it takes a team of the right people to pull these together for effective outcomes.

- Learn from other families and from other health care teams about what works. What has been tried that should be avoided? For example, health system improvement specialists are looking to reduce the isolation in approaches to health care, making it less "siloed". Yet many programs install care coordinators in an old model that continues to foster isolation and without thought to family-centered, team based, quality improvement. Care coordinators can be instrumental in systems development, tests of improvement and fostering an integrated system.

(3) Be true to pediatrics. Children are not young adults. At times it seems that this old lesson has been forgotten. As the medical home gains traction, many lessons learned and reform initiatives are grounded in adult care. This can be an opportunity for the spread of medical home innovation; it can also be a frustration for pediatric focused teams who are asked to use adult based approaches in their system of care. Advocacy is needed for systems and services designed to partner with children and families for success, and for the professionals who specialize in how to build these healing relationships.

(4) Seek the "win win". As a team you may be looking for strategies to help you—improve care delivery while tracking progress and performance; enhance teamwork with strong involvement of families; partner well across systems; engage children and families in their care; connect families to one another for support; frame the role responsibilities of a care coordinator; or find ways to motivate and empower families and staff. Shared care-planning and the use of shared care plans described above touches on most of these targets and does so with one intervention targeting multiple goals rather than eight different initiatives. See Fig. 5.2 "Win-wins" are efficient, effective and energizing; shared care planning with shared plans of care offers a win-win innovation.

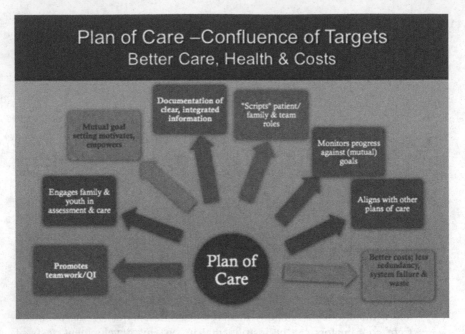

Fig. 5.2 A confluence of targets or "win-win" approach

5.7 Summary

This chapter suggests some concepts from the literature which can be used to scaffold learning towards the development and delivery of family-centered care coordination. There is shared foundational knowledge ready for use; there is also new work such as jointly created and shared plans of care that need to be tested and improved upon. A primary goal of care coordination is how to best learn from and partner with families. This chapter suggests that forming a highly functioning improvement team who will work towards ongoing care innovations is an important step to securing effective family-centered care coordination. Such a team searches for ways to integrate and make sense of information so that it can be useful for all team members and particularly families whose children live with special health care needs. Shared care-planning offers a strategy for teams to use in creating better care and more effective systems of care. Individual children and families are engaged to help summarize critical information, set goals, negotiate actions, clarifying accountabilities and carry out plans together with clear support and oversight. Improvement teams learn continuously from one another; they also learn from other individual patients and families. This is all about how to make care and care coordination better. In the words of Kenneth Blanchard, "None of us is as smart as all of us". Care coordination and now Shared Care-Planning opens the door for the combined effect of all partners to be captured as a consensus approach using a jointly created plan of care. These plans are used and improved upon to better the quality of life of children with special health care needs and their families on a daily basis.

References

McPherson, M., et al. (1998). A new definition of children with special health care needs. *Pediatrics, 102*(1 Pt 1), 137–140.

American Academy of Pediatrics Commitee on Children with Disabilities (2005). Care coordination in the medical home: Integrating health and related systems of care for children with special health care needs. *Pediatrics, 116*(5), 1238–1244.

American Academy of Pediatrics Medical Home Initiatives for Children With Special Needs Project Advisory Committee (2008). The medical home. *Pediatrics*, 2002, *110*(1), 184–186 (Reaffirmed 2008).

Antonelli, R. C., Stille, C. J., & Antonelli, D. M. (2008). Care coordination for children and youth with special health care needs: A descriptive, multisite study of activities, personnel costs and outcomes. *Pediatrics, 122*(1), 209–216.

Antonelli, R., McAllister, J., & Popp, J. (2009). *Making care coordination a critical component of the pediatric health care system: A multidisciplinary framework.* The Commonwealth Fund: New York.

Cooley, W. C., & McAllister, J. W. (2004). Building Medical Homes: Improvement Strategies in Primary Care for Children with Special Health Care Needs. *Pediatrics (Supplement), 113*, 1499–1506.

Looman, W. S., Presler, E., Erickson, M. M., Garwick, A. W., Cady, R. G., Kelly, A. M., et al. (2013) Care coordination for children with complex special health care needs: The value of the advanced practice Nurse's enhanced scope of knowledge and practice. *Journal of Pediatric Health Care, 27*(4), 293–303.

Nutting, P. A., et al. (2009). Initial lessons from the first national demonstration project on practice transformation to a patient-centered medical home. *Annals of Family Medicine, 7*(3), 254–260.

McAllister, J. W., et al. (2013). Medical home transformation in pediatric primary care–what drives change? *Annals of Family Medicine, 11*(Suppl 1), S90–S98.

McAllister, J., et al. (2014) *Achieving a shared plan of care for children and youth with special health care needs.* Lucille Packard Foundation for Children's Healthcare: Lucille Packard Foundation for Children's Healthcare (in press).

McAllister, J. (2014) *Achieving a shared plan of care for children and youth with special health care needs: A learning guide.* Lucille Packard Foundation for Children's Healthcare: Lucille Packard Foundation for Children's Healthcare (in press).

National Center for Medical Home implementation (2014). Retrieved July 1, from http://www.medicalhomeinfo.org/

Strickland, B., McPherson, M., Weissman, G., van Dyck, P., Huang, Z. J., & Newacheck, P. (2004). Access to the medical home: Results of the National Survey of Children with Special Health Care Needs. *Pediatrics, 113*(5), 1485–1492.

Stille, C. J., & Antonelli, R. C. (2004). Coordination of care for children with special health care needs. *Current Opinion in Pediatrics, 16*, 700–705, Retrieved from http://journals.lww.com/copediatrics/pages/default.aspx

Chapter 6
Transitional Care Management

6.1 Case Management, Care Coordination and Transition

The terms care management, case management and care coordination are beginning to receive the recognition they so rightfully deserve, though the terms have been around for decades. The phrase "care coordination," as a role associated with transitional care, is spoken by a number of individuals including legislators and regulators in Washington D.C.; leaders of both payer and provider systems; case management professional colleagues; and patients who were previously lost in complex and often confusing healthcare system. The phrase is found 14 times in the Accountable Care Act. The interest in care transitions is causing policy makers, care providers, advocacy groups, and families to want a measurement of how well entities do in care transition. As an example from a hospital perspective, patient satisfaction surveys—commonly identified as the Hospital Consumer Assessment of Hospital Providers and Systems—for 2014 are anticipated to include the following care transitions measures (Centers for Medicare and Medicaid 2013a, b):

- The hospital staff took my preferences and those of my family into account when deciding what my health care needs would be when I left the hospital.
- When I left the hospital, I had a good understanding of the things I was responsible for in managing my health.
- When I left the hospital, I clearly understood the purpose for taking each of my medications.

So exactly what is transitional care management and why the increased interest in it? Fundamentally transition of care or care transitions, is the movement of patients from one health care practitioner or setting to another as their condition and care needs change. Care transitions can occur within a setting (intensive care to medical surgical floor); between setting (acute care to skilled nursing facility);

© The Author(s) 2015   61
J. Treadwell et al., *Case Management and Care Coordination*,
SpringerBriefs in Child Health, DOI 10.1007/978-3-319-07224-1_6

across health states (curative care to hospice); or across health providers (pediatric to adult setting). The majority of studies and work related to care transitions have focused on the elderly, as they are a population with complex care needs, including admissions and readmissions. However, transitional care program development may be applied to all populations and is increasingly being seen in advanced in research (Taylor et al. 2013). One specific area of interest has been in the safe discharge transition of infants from the neonatal intensive care unit (NICU) and the coordination and education needed to prevent readmissions and gain compliance with a first pediatrician visit (Moyer et al. 2010).

6.2 Policy Momentum and History

The Committee on Healthcare Quality in America, formed by the Institute of Medicine, investigated quality of care beginning over 15 years ago. This Committee's initial report, *Crossing the Quality Chasm* provided a concerning and comprehensive review of the overall quality of the health care system, including an assessment of its safety and effectiveness and recommendations for a comprehensive strategy for improvement (Institute of Medicine 2001). The Committee still exists today with one of their concerns being safe and efficient care transitions. In 2031, they have additionally formed a subcommittee on Improving the Health, Safety, and Well-Being of Young Adults (age 18–26) due to the issues of chronic condition care and lack of access to health care, exacerbated by poor transition to the adult care community, placing these individuals at risk, or vulnerable to poor health care outcomes (http://www.iom.edu/Activities/Children/ImprovingYoungAdultHealth. aspx).

> Tip for Families: Ask the case manager at your child's hospital to explain what measures they have in place to ensure a successful discharge without readmission? Do they offer a home visit to support medication reconciliation?

> Tip for Health Care Professional: Making sure that communication from hospitalists and specialists occurs at discharge with the receiving community pediatrician requires a solid protocol. Make sure to connect with the hospital case management department and are informed of the communication protocol in effect.

Section 3025 of the Affordable Care Act added Section 1886(q) to the Social Security Act establishing the Hospital Readmissions Reduction Program (http:// www.cms.gov/Medicare/Medicare-Fee-for-Service-Payment/AcuteInpatientPPS/ FY-2012-IPPS-Final-Rule-Home-Page-Items/CMS1250103.html), which requires CMS to reduce payments to inpatient prospective payment system (IPPS) hospitals with excess readmissions, effective for discharges beginning on October 1, 2012. CMS has also established an Improving Care Transitions program in Medicaid. The recognition that transitions between care settings is critical to improving outcomes, and quality of care has initiated a Program focus on transition issues of:

- Preventing medical errors;
- Identification of issues for early intervention;
- Preventing unnecessary hospitalizations and readmissions;
- Supporting family preferences and choices; and
- Avoiding duplication of services and efforts.

Care coordination was defined to be necessary in the coordination of medical and long term supports and services (LTSS) when an individual is:

- Admitted to a hospital, emergency room, or other for acute medical care;
- Discharged from a hospital to an institutional long term care (LTC) setting, such as a skilled nursing facility/nursing facility (SNF/NF), inpatient rehabilitation facility (IRF), or intermediate care facility (ICF);
- Discharged to community based LTC; or
- Discharged from an institutional LTC care setting to community LTC or vice versa.

http://www.medicaid.gov/Medicaid-CHIP-Program-Information/By-Topics/Quality-of-Care/Care-Transitions.html

In April 2011, CMS announced the development of the Community-Based Care Transition Program (http://innovation.cms.gov/initiatives/CCTP) created by Section 3026 of the Patient Protection and Affordable Care Act (PPACA). The CCTP provides funding opportunities for acute-care hospitals with high readmission rates that partner with community based organizations (CBOs). This initiative is part of the Partnership for Patients, a public public-private partnership charged with reducing hospital-acquired conditions by 40 % and hospital readmissions by 20 % by 2013. The Department of Health and Human Services agreed to invest up to $1 billion in PPACA funds in the Partnership to reduce millions of preventable injuries and complications. There are currently 102 organizations participating in the CCTP. Participants will use process and outcome measures to report on their results. Multiple studies have shown there are many factors along the care continuum that impact readmissions, and identifying the key drivers of readmissions for a hospital and its downstream providers is the first step towards implementing the appropriate interventions necessary for reducing readmissions for patients of all ages. The Hospital Readmissions Reduction Program and the Improving Care Transitions Program has potentially significant financial impacts for hospitals and has caused an increase in attention on the development of transitional care management programs in an attempt to reduce hospital readmission rates.

6.3   Organizational Development and Research

A professional initiative of The Case Management Society of America (www.cmsa.org) and Sanofi-aventis U.S. LLC announced on October 3, 2006, the establishment of the National Transitions of Care Coalition (www.ntocc.org) to improve the quality of care between health care settings, particularly for seniors. This joint project addresses filling the gaps that occur when patients leave one care setting and move to another care setting. Transitions include children moving from primary care to specialty physicians; moving or transferring children from the emergency department to intensive care or surgery; or when patients are discharged from the hospital to home, assisted living arrangements or skilled nursing facilities. Care transitions ensure the needs and preferences for health services through information sharing across people, functions, and sites of care over time. Care transitions must be embraced by organizations, not individuals. It is truly a team effort with the focus on patient goals and preferences. Every care coordination team needs to have a culture of trust, shared goals, effective communication and mutual respect for different skill contributions and roles of each team member. Care transition is a process, not an event. Transitions are provider hand-OVER, not hand-OFF.

The U.S. health care system often fails to meet the needs of vulnerable populations during transitions because care is rushed and responsibility is fragmented, with little communication across care settings or among providers. A burden is placed on children/families in initiating their follow-up care with little understanding of their conditions or the complexities of today's health care system. There is increasing awareness among health care professionals and government leaders that the U.S. health care system must focus efforts on improving the coordination of care among the various care settings to improve patient safety, quality of care and outcomes. The focus of the National Transitions of Care Coalition (NTOCC) is to bring together thought leaders and health care participants from various settings to address this critical issue. The NTOCC attempts to find solutions and develops tools to address the gaps impacting safety and the quality of care for transitioning patients, particularly seniors, and makes these tools available to the health care industry.

NTOCC was initially started by thirteen leading national health care industry organizations. The initial meeting was held on October 18, 2006, in Chicago, Illinois. Participating groups included the American Society on Aging, the American Geriatrics Society, the American Society of Health System Pharmacists Research and Education Foundation, the American College of Healthcare Executives, the American Society of Consultant Pharmacists, the Institute of Healthcare Improvement, the Case Management Society of America, the Joint Commission International Center for Patient Safety, the Roger C. Lipitz Center for Integrated Health Care, the Mid-America Coalition on Health Care, the National Association of Social Workers, sanofi-aventis U.S. LLC, the Society of Hospital Medicine, and URAC. The participants agreed that transitions of care is a major issue in the United States and can only be solved by breaking down the silos and barriers between different health care settings and working collaboratively for the good of the patient.

The NTOCC wanted to build awareness among legislators and policymakers that the following considerations should be part of any health care reform initiative:

- Improve communication during transitions between providers, patients, and caregivers;
- Implement electronic medical records that include standardized medication reconciliation elements;
- Establish points of accountability for sending and receiving care, particularly for hospitalists, SNFists, primary care physicians, and specialists;
- Increase the use of case management and professional care coordination;
- Expand the role of the pharmacist in transitions of care;
- Implement payment systems that align incentives; and
- Develop performance measures to encourage better transitions of care.

The NTOCC work groups developed a set of tools and resources that were piloted and released to the public in April 2008. The tools represent the culmination of several months of collaboration between twenty-nine industry stakeholders to address the challenges associated with transitions of care. The NTOCC also released accompanying information on how to implement and measure the tools, as well as material designed to raise industry, policymaker, media, and the general public's awareness of transitions of care. The material is available on the NTOCC website (http://www.ntocc.org/WhoWeServe/HealthCareProfessionals. aspx). The tools were developed to help health care professionals, organizations, and patients address problems inherent in transitioning patients from one level of care to another.

In July 2009, the NTOCC formed the Health Information Technology Work Group. The work group focuses on the national efforts to develop electronic medical records, health information technology (HIT) exchange, and promote interoperability to advance improved patient care. The work group's activities included assessment of the barriers and gaps in HIT related to transitions of care (TOC) and the development of a white paper that would provide recommendations on how to close gaps or remove barriers (http://www.ntocc.org/News/tabid/59/ month/8/year/2009/Default.aspx).

6.4 Tools and Application

One of the most logical and useful tools to assist families and case managers in successful transitions is the *Ask Me Three*™ program developed by Partnership for Clear Health Communication at the National Patient Safety Foundation. Smooth discharges begin at the time of admission. Providing children and caregivers with the proper tools early in the admission will help to ensure a better transition to the next level of care. The program encourages families to ask their healthcare providers the following three questions and write down the answers:

- What is my (child's) main problem? This helps patients and families better understand the diagnosis.
- What do I (child/family) need to do? Helps better understand the plan of care.

- Why is it important for me (child/family) to do this? Helps with internal motivation.

Source: http://www.pfizerhealthliteracy.com/physicians-providers/PchcAskme3. aspx

As simple as this seems, these questions can cause increased communication about the plan of care that clarify misconceptions which could lead to error or injury. Case managers are instrumental in coaching patients, caregivers, and family to take an active role in care transitions. Asking questions of healthcare professionals is a great start for families to take an active role in the care coordination team. The University of Texas Health Science Center at San Antonio conducted a study where they evaluated use of Ask Me 3 in a pediatric health center. The results showed every parent (n = 393, 31 % Spanish speaking) felt the program was beneficial in getting them more information (Mika et al. 2007). Patients and families don't always feel comfortable voicing concerns and questions. The same holds true for verbalizing preferences. It is important for case mangers to encourage patient and families to actively participate in the care plan and remind patients and families that they have the right to the following:

- Be treated fairly and with respect during care transitions.
- Know why a care transition is needed.
- Verbalize preferences during care transitions.
- Take part in planning care transitions.
- Know the costs related to care transitions.
- Know the people and organizations involved in the care transitions.
- Know the next steps during care transitions.
- Privacy of health care information during care transitions.
- Where to go for assistance when care transitions don't go well.

Tips for Parents:

- Determine your primary point of contact in a healthcare setting and keep the lines of communication open. It is OK to speak your mind and disagree with the proposed plan of care if it does not meet your needs.
- Speak up and ask questions-it is OK to seek clarification and there truly is no "dumb" question.
- Realize that the decisions on how to proceed with care are yours to make. You are in the driver seat and your desires and preferences should be incorporated into the plan of care.

Tips for Healthcare Professionals:

- Understand your role in the care continuum-do you have the information you need for the patient's upcoming appointment?
- Communicate openly and honestly with patients and family so they can make informed decisions.

- Really listen to patients and family to determine preferences that must be included in the plan of care.
- Never assume anything-ask questions regardless of how basic to ensure the patient has adequate knowledge of the plan of care and the support systems to implement the plan.

Case Managers can support families in transitions across care setting or practitioners by informing families on choices, providing tools for reminders, and linking families with resources. All of these things help build competency in the family to identify issues of safety and continuity which might impact care outcomes. Engaging the family to begin the process is often the most difficult task. Providing families with a tangible resource and timeline, in the form of an online tool or care binder, may act as a catalyst to begin planning. way to connect patients, families, and providers with services and resources to support coordinated, continuous care (Taylor et al. 2013).

Case managers are most often responsible for TCM and should have proficiency in chronic disease management, motivational interviewing, and behavioral change theory to successfully fulfill this role. Home visits are increasing in TCM programs, with 60 % of the survey respondents noting they provide home visits for certain patients.

In developing a transitional care program, it is important to include the key concepts of:

- Shift from the concept of "discharge" to "transfer with continuous management".
- Begin transfer planning upon or before admission.
- Review past medical history and previous admissions, and identify potential reasons for readmission.
- Ensure the patient is stable for transfer or discharge.
- Ensure the patient and caregiver understands the purpose of the transfer or discharge.
- Incorporate the patient's and caregiver's preferences into the transitional plan.
- Identify the patient's social and caregiver support.
- Collaborate with practitioners across settings to formulate and execute a common care plan.
- Ensure the receiving provider is capable and prepared (if applicable).
- For transfers, ensure that the care plan, orders, and a clinical summary precede the patient's arrival. The receiving provider should clarify discrepancies regarding the care plan, the patient's status, or the patient's medications.
- Focus on medical and behavioral health integration. Many chronic illnesses have behavioral health components.
- For discharges, ensure the patient has a timely follow-up appointment.
- One area of transition extremely important to families with Children with Special Health.

6.5 Adolescent Transition to Adult Care

Care coordination requires special attention for Children with Special Healthcare Needs (CSHCN) in transitioning from pediatric practitioners to adult care providers.

Adolescent transition requires the care coordination team to identify quality providers that will deliver developmentally appropriate services to provide care continuity. The case manager role is to develop an individualized plan to move from pediatric to adult care. Since the active transition ideally occurs between the ages of 18 and 21 years, initial planning begins at age 14 where, as capable, the adolescent begins to become increasingly involved and set expectations for selecting and understanding how to navigate in an adult healthcare environment. Coordinating adolescent transition as a family and healthcare team supports youth as they move to assume adult roles, which includes managing their health (Cooley and Sagerman 2011).

> Tips for HealthCare Professionals: to assess if your practice is delivering appropriate transition care, perform a practice-evaluation. A good tool to use is the *Medical Home Health Care Transition Index for Youth Up to Age 18* which can be found at: http://www. gottransition.org/UploadedFiles/Files/8_CMHI_HCT_Index_Pediatric_09NOV2011_.pdf.

Finding adult practitioners may not be an easy task. The majority of adult internal medicine providers are not comfortable providing primary care for young adults with chronic illnesses. Researching what providers are amenable to caring for CSHCN, can be initially researched telephonically however, a test of practice style and acceptable communication style and comfort is important to arrange through office visits occurring prior to the termination of pediatric care relationships. Efforts to increase familiarity in residency programs with care needs of CSHCN, or creating specialty just-in-time consulting for existing medical homes, are strategies that shows promise in creating improved comfort of providers, and therefore healthcare access for the young adults with complex chronic conditions (Okumura et al. 2008).

References

American Academy of Pediatrics. (2002, December). American Academy of Family Physicians; American College of Physicians–American Society of Internal Medicine. A consensus statement on health care transitions for young adults with special health care needs. *Pediatrics, 110*(6 Pt 2), 1304–1306.

Centers for Medicare and Medicaid Services. (2013a). *HCAHPS Training Update*. Center for Medicare. Retrieved from http://www.hcahpsonline.org/Files/March%202013%20HCAHPS %20Update%20Training%20Slides_3-6-13.pdf.

Centers for Medicare and Medicaid Services. (2013b). Improving care transitions. Retrieved from http://www.medicaid.gov/Medicaid-CHIP-Program-Information/By-Topics/Quality-of-Care/ Care-Transitions.html.

Cooley, W., & Sagerman, P. (2011, July). American Academy of Physicians; American Academy of Family Physicians; American College of Physicians; transitions clinical report authoring group. Supporting the health care transition from adolescence to adulthood in the medical home. *Pediatrics, 1*, 182–200. doi:10.1542/peds.2011-0969. Retrieved from http://pediatrics. aappublications.org/content/128/1/182.full.

Institute of Medicine. (2001, March). *Crossing the Quality Chasm.* National Academies. Retrieved from http://www.iom.edu/Reports/2001/Crossing-the-Quality-Chasm-A-New-Health-System-for-the-21st-Century.asp.

Mika, V., Wood, P., Weis, B., & Trevino, L. (2007). Ask Me 3; improving communication in a Hispanic pediatric outpatient practice. *American Journal of Health Behavior, S1*, 115–121.

Moyer, V., Singh, H., Finfel, K., & Giardino, A. (2010). Transitions from neonatal intensive care unit to ambulatory care: description and evaluation of the proactive risk assessment process. *Quality and Safety in Health Care, 19*, i26–i30. doi:10.1136/qshc.2010.040543.

Okumura, M., Heisler, M., Davis, M., Cabana, M., Demonner, S., & Kerr, E. (2008, October). Comfort of general internists and general pediatricians in providing care for young adults with chronic illnesses of childhood. *Journal of General Internal Medicine, 23*(10):1621–1627. doi:10.1007/s11606-008-0716-8.

Taylor, A., Lizzi, M., Marx, A., Chilkatowsky, M., Trachtenberg, S., & Ogle, S. (2013, September). Implementing a care coordination program for children with special healthcare needs: partnering with families and providers. *Journal of Healthcare Quality, 35*(5),70–77. doi:10.1111/j.1945-1474.

Chapter 7
Home Visitation and Care Coordination

7.1 Home Visitation Programs: Definition

Home visitation is defined as a process by which health services are provided to a family in its own home over a sustained period of time (Wasik et al. 1990). The practice of visiting families in the home is based on the assumptions that parents are the most important people in the lives of children and the home is the most important setting for children. The goal of home visitation is to help parents enhance the child's development by providing support and knowledge. However, in order for the parents to respond effectively to their children, attention has to also be focused on their own needs. Parents who are concerned about basic needs such as housing or food, or who are affected by other stressors, will have a hard time caring for their children (Wasik et al. 1990). In this regard, the goals of home visitation and case management are fundamentally synergetic as both include longitudinal and comprehensive interventions with parents to promote the health and well-being of the family. Thus, the home visitor's role in delivering comprehensive care to families is consistent with the role of a case manager who mobilizes resources to address the multiple needs of children and families.

Home visitation programs have been implemented in the United States since the 19th century as a way to address the health care needs of women and children (Weiss 1993). Public health nurses, social workers, or other trained staff provided ongoing in-home health education to women and children, primarily in urban settings. This approach to health care continued in the 20th century where the focus was on families with special needs such as premature or low birth-weight infants, children with developmental delays, and teenage parents. The accumulating evidence about the potential benefits of home visitation programs prompted the Council on Child and Adolescent Health to later endorse home visitation programs as an effective way to improve health outcomes for children and families (American Academy of Pediatrics 1998). The American Academy of Pediatrics encourages pediatricians to recognize that home visitation programs can

© The Author(s) 2015
J. Treadwell et al., *Case Management and Care Coordination*,
SpringerBriefs in Child Health, DOI 10.1007/978-3-319-07224-1_7

supplement office- based care and be part of Medical Home concept that provides a continuum of care. Pediatricians are encouraged to support referrals of high-risk parents to home visitation programs as early as possible. Suggestions are also made for advocacy in order to support funding for quality home visitation programs.

Family Tip
Access to a Home Visitation Program may be offered by the health care provider or can be obtained by contacting the member services number on the health insurance card. The Affordable Care Act in 2010 allocated $1.5 billion to expand home visitation programs in the United States so most likely these programs are available in your community.

Healthcare Professional Tip
Health care professionals can refer families to home visitations program by contacting the individual's health plan or identifying other programs in the community.

7.2 Models of Home Visitation Programs

There are many maternal, infant and early child models of home visitation programs that are implemented across the United States. The U.S. Department of Health and Human Services has identified several home visitation programs with evidence of effectiveness (U.S. Department of Health and Human Services 2013). These programs vary in their focus but they all involve regular home visits by paraprofessionals, social workers or nurses. Some of the more known programs include the following:

Healthy Families America (HFA). HFA is a national evidence-based program in 40 states, District of Colombia, and all five US territories that works with families beginning during prenatal care and can extend as long as three to five years after the child has been born. Paraprofessionals implement the program based on three critical program elements: service initiation, service content, and staff characteristics. These home visits, which are conducted on a weekly to biweekly schedule, focus on supporting parents, the child-parent interactions and educating parents to prevent child maltreatment (Healthy Families America 2014).

Nurse Family Partnership (NFP). NFP is a program for first time, low income mothers that has been implemented in 32 states. This program is delivered by registered nurses who create a foundation for strong families by supporting the mothers and encouraging them to have a healthy pregnancy. The registered nurse visits the home once a week for the first month then taper to biweekly until the child is born. For the first six weeks after the child is born, visits resume to weekly and then continue biweekly until the child is approximately twenty months old. Leading up to the child's second birthday, there are four final visits that occur monthly (Nurse-Family Partnership 2014).

Healthy Start. Healthy Start programs, which are implemented in 38 states, the District of Columbia and Puerto Rico, focus on at-risk families during the first year of the infant's life (National Healthy Start Association 2014). This program is delivered by paraprofessionals who address parent-child interactions and identify a reliable support figure for the child. The intensity of home visitation vary in frequency of visits depending on the client (McCurdy 2005).

Early Head Start. Early Head Start is a federal program that has been implemented in all 50 states, the District of Columbia, Puerto Rico and the U.S. Virgin Islands. This program focuses on child development, family development, community building and staff development in low income families with infants and toddlers, and pregnant women and their families. There are four different program options: center-based services, home-based services, family child care services, and combination services which include both home and center based services. On average, the home-based services include a visit from a paraprofessional twice per month to deliver the child-focused program to help the parents support their child's development (Love et al. 2005).

Parents as Teachers. Parents as Teachers program is being utilized in all 50 states and six other countries. This program focuses on preventing child abuse, providing a solid foundation for school success for children, giving parents the tools to increase knowledge of child development and fostering growth and learning, and develop home-school-community partnerships (Parents as Teachers 2014). This program has monthly regularly scheduled home visits by certified parent educators, parent group meetings, periodic developmental screenings and referrals to community services. The target populations of this program are parents and their children (beginning prenatally and continuing until the child is three to five years of age), parents who are teenagers, and parents whose children attend child care centers (Wagner et al. 2002).

All of the home visiting programs involve at-risk families and seek to foster a better child-parent bond. With the exception of the Healthy Start program, all other four programs begin with prenatal patients. While the frequency of the program and the deliverer of the program vary, they all have the same fundamental focus on the relationship between the parent and child in order to create an environment where the parents feel better equipped to care for and nurture their child.

Other home visitation programs that are also part of the U.S. Department of Health and Human Services include Child FIRST, Early Intervention Program for Adolescent Mothers, Early Start (New Zealand), Family Check-Up, Healthy Steps, Home Instruction for Parents of Preschool Youngsters (HIPPY), Oklahoma Community-Based Family Resource and Support Program, and Play and Learning Strategies (PALS) (U.S. Department of Health and Human Services 2013).

Family Tip
Several Home Visitation Programs may be available in the community. Consult a health care provider about the best fit for the patient and the family. Some of the programs are available based on a geographic area.

Healthcare Professional Tip
Several Home Visitation programs may be in the community. Become familiar with the focus of these programs to ensure the best fit for your patients.

7.3 Evidence of the Benefits of Home Visitation

Several reviews of the literature were conducted to examine evidence about the
effectiveness of home visitation programs in improving maternal) and child outcomes. For example, a review of prenatal home visiting programs was conducted
to determine the effectiveness of prenatal home visitation for improving prenatal
care utilization and preventing preterm birth and low birth weight (Issel et al.
2011). The review included 28 studies comparing outcomes of women who
received prenatal home visiting with women who did not. Fourteen of the studies
used a randomized controlled design. Another systematic review evaluated the
effectiveness of paraprofessional home visitation programs in improving developmental and health outcomes of children from disadvantaged families (Peacock
et al. 2013). The review included 21 randomized controlled trials. A systematic
review of studies was also conducted to examine evidence regarding home visitation and outcomes of preterm births (Goyal et al. 2013). The review included 17
studies of which 15 were randomized controlled trials. The reviews have documented the following outcomes:

Prenatal Effects

- Improvement in prenatal care utilization
- Positive effect on gestational age
- Positive effect on birth weight

Postnatal Effects

- Increase in psychomotor and cognitive development
- Increase in birth weight
- Increase in developmental outcomes
- Increase in positive parent-infant interaction
- Increase in weight and height during infancy

Long Term Effects

- Decrease in reported child abuse
- Decrease in health problems in older children
- Increase in language skills

Overall, studies support that home visitation programs promote parent-child
interaction, utilization of prenatal care, and developmental and health outcomes of
young children from disadvantaged families. However, some studies did not
document statistically significant benefits, especially in the area of child abuse and
neglect. Additionally, the reviewers identify common methodological limitations
such as limited sample size, high attrition rates that may have contributed to
biases, and lack of statistical information to allow a meta-analysis. Further studies
using rigorous designs and measures including program intensity, are needed to
examine the role of home visitation in improving maternal and child outcomes.

Family Tip
Discuss with the health care provider the best Home Visitation to select from the programs
that are available in the patient/patient family's community. Information can be requested
to help make an informed decision.

Healthcare Professional Tip
Become familiar with the outcomes of Home Visitation programs and support referrals to
programs that were adequately evaluated and have documented evidence for improving
outcomes. Be willing to participate in evaluating these programs in your community.

7.4   Elements of Successful Home Visitation Programs

Several essential elements have been identified as effective in improving home
visitation outcomes (Olds 1992; Peacock et al. 2013). This includes the following:

(1) A focus on families at greater need for the services as opposed to universal
     programs;
(2) Interventions that begin during pregnancy and continue follow-up at least
     through the second year of the child's life;
(3) Promotion of positive health-related behaviors and qualities of infant care
     giving;
(4) Provisions to reduce family stress by improving the social and physical
     environments in which families live;
(5) Tailoring services to address the family's specific needs and risk level
(6) The program needs to focus on addressing the multiple problems that affect
     the family, and
(7) Those who are helping the families need to be trained adequately to meet the
     needs of those they are serving.

7.5   Client-Home Visitor Alliance

The development of a trusting and supportive relationship between the home
visitor and the family is crucial for effective care. The importance of these relationships is well documented in nursing and social work research. Approaches to
relationship development have been described on a continuum from professional-
centered to family-centered and are based on assumptions about family competencies and the relationships that professionals form with families (Dunst et al.
1991). Family-centered practices include relational and participatory aspects. The
relational aspect includes good clinical skills such as listening, compassion,
empathy, respect, and being non-judgmental and professional beliefs about parenting capabilities and competencies. The participatory component includes
practices that are individualized, flexible and responsive to the family's needs, and

provide opportunities for the family to be actively engaged in making decisions to achieve desired goals. Family-centered approaches are those that employ relational and participatory components.

7.6 Home Visitation Challenges

7.6.1 Program Attrition

Attrition is a significant challenge for a home visitation program as it reduces its effectiveness (Raikes et al. 2006). Attrition occurs when the clients no longer desire to stay in the program or when they cannot be reached for scheduling meetings. For example, only 35 to 40 % of participants remained engaged in NFP sites (O'Brien et al. 2012). Holland et al. (2014) identify in their review of studies several factors that can contribute to program attrition. Factors reported by clients include busy lifestyle with competing priorities, a low perceived need for the services, and sufficient social support. Factors identified by home visitors included difficulties in reaching the clients for scheduling, family loss of interest in the program, and the family moving away. A recent qualitative study using semi structured interviews and focus groups with mothers who dropped out of the NFP programs were conducted (Holland et al. 2014). Of 196 mothers contacted, 21 (11 %) were successfully interviewed. Participants also included eight nurses and three nurse supervisors. Barriers identified by mothers included busy schedules and being overwhelmed by other responsibilities, unstable and crowded housing conditions, nurses did not meet expectations, program content was not relevant, decreased interest in program after the child was born, family intrusion, difficulty communicating with NFP, and leaving the area for an extended period of time. The authors conclude that retention can be improved by ensuring the program addresses the individual needs of the mothers and help mothers increase organizational and communication skills.

7.6.2 Program Fidelity

As evidence of the benefits of home visitation programs has been established, a focus on program fidelity has emerged. While program fidelity is important to ensure consistent implementation, some concerns were raised in programs such as NFP about the ability of protocol-directed care to allow nurses to respond to the specific needs of clients (Zeanah et al. 2006). It is asserted that relational and ethical knowledge and skills used by nurses as well as client perspectives cannot be fully integrated in protocols (Strom et al. 2011). Smithbattle et al. (2013) have implemented and evaluated *Listening with Care*, a home visiting intervention utilizing narrative methods and therapeutic tools to train nurses on strengthening responsive relationships with teen mothers. Nurses were trained to use clinical interviews to foster effective listening, express the baby's needs, develop baby book journals from the baby's perspective, and therapeutic letter writing to patients between encounters to reinforce clinical progress. The evaluation included a quasi-experimental design that examined the effect of the intervention on depressive symptoms, self-resiliency, repeat pregnancy, and educational progress among pregnant teens participating in the home visiting program compared to pregnant teens who did not participate in such a program. Qualitative data were collected from the perspectives of the nurses to assess the feasibility and acceptability of the intervention. The results of the study indicated that nurses endorsed the intervention and felt that the therapeutic tools encouraged them to listen to the teens and broadened their understanding of the teens' lives. The study did not find statistical significant differences between the groups on maternal outcomes. The authors believe that feedback from teens and nurses emphasize the importance of attentive care that may not be provided in programs that emphasize fidelity to protocols.

7.6.3 Home Visitation Safety

Neighborhoods that have high crime and violence rates are also those that are the most in need for home visitation (Nadwairski 1992). This presents a major issue related to the safety of the home visitors. A qualitative study was conducted with administrators and staff from home health agencies in order to better understand personal safety risk issues facing home health staff (Fazzone et al. 2000). The study included focus groups, in-depth individual interviews, and critical event narratives. Staff identified organizational and administrative issues that could impede personal safety. This included absence of written policies and procedures about safety, polices that were not enforced, lack of administrative support, and staff and administrators unfamiliarity with the community. The study also identified certain protective factors that helped keep staff safe. This included characteristics such as self-confidence, self-reliance, self-motivation, flexibility, and self-assurance about personal judgment. In light of the findings, the authors recommend that home visitation programs implement ongoing education and training and that policies and procedures are developed and reviewed with staff several times a year. This is needed as safety concerns can affect the staff and compromise patient care.

To address home visitation safety, many established programs have developed comprehensive personal safety policies and procedures. These manuals address safety in three categories: before the visit, approaching the house, and during the visit. Before the visit, home visitors are guided to make sure they are wearing comfortable clothes and dressing appropriately. They should inform the program about the visit and carry a cell phone in case of emergencies. When approaching the house, the visitors are advised to be aware of their surroundings, parking the vehicle in a strategic place for a quick exit, and locking valuables in the car. During the visit, the visitors are advised to be in a position at all times where the exit can be accessed. Some samples of guidelines can be accessed for more details (Nurse Family Partnership's Home Visiting Service Guide, Healthy Families America Site Development Guide).

7.6.4 Ethical Considerations

Prevention of child maltreatment has been a significant focus for home visiting programs and has been evaluated as a program outcome (Olds et al. 1995). Issues surrounding mandated reporting of child abuse and maltreatment are pertinent to nurses working in home visitation settings. Nurse home visitors who visit their clients at home may encounter instances of suspected child abuse and maltreatment. As health care professionals, nurses are trained on child abuse reporting requirements and are mandated to report these cases. Nurses may be concerned about reporting as it may harm their relationship with the client. However, if a nurse does not contact authorities when she encounters reportable child abuse instances, she may face legal ramifications for failure to report. Coupled with the home visitors' supportive roles is a legal mandate to report instances of child maltreatment to child protective services. Training about maltreatment reporting procedures in home visitation programs with local child protective service agencies to determine reporting requirements will reduce ambiguity and increase competency.

7.6.5 Health Literacy

Health literacy, defined as the ability to access, understand, and use health information to promote health, has been associated with a variety of health promoting behaviors in adults and children (Davis et al. 2013). Parental health literacy is critical for engaging families in decision making to support health promotion activities for children. Knowledge on the family's capacity to understand and carry out health-related tasks, and tailoring the messages to the appropriate literacy level is crucial. Health literacy is important in home visitation programs as very often the populations targeted is at risk for low health literacy (Weiss 1993). Smith and Moore (2012) studied 2,572 parent/child dyads who participated in one of seven home visitation programs in five states to examine the development of health literacy among parents. The selected programs (Healthy Families America, National Healthy Start, Early Head Start, Parents as Teaches, Strengthening Families, CHIP of Virginia, and a telephonic case management model for families in rural areas in New Mexico), have a specific focus on promoting health literacy and developing reflective functioning among parents. Significant improvements have been seen in management of personal and child health when participants improved their health literacy. The study showed that a reflective model of home visitation can empower parents to better manage personal and child health and healthcare. For parents to be engaged in the health of their children, they must be provided information they understand and can use to care for their children (Davis et al. 2013). A family-centered approach that recognizes and respect families' unique differences has been shown to improve health, nutrition, safety, parenting, and psychosocial issues.

Family Tip
If there is concern about the relationships with the home visitor or she is not responsive to needs, make sure to talk about it with the program's supervisor. A supervisor will be able to identify a different home visitor who may be a better fit.

Healthcare Professional Tip
The relationships you form with the clients are crucial for program success. Family-centered approaches that include listening, compassion, empathy, and respect are the most effective. It is also important to ensure that you are responsive to the client's needs.

References

American Academy of Pediatrics, Council on Child and Adolescent Health. (1998). The role of home-visitation programs in improving health outcomes for children and families. *Pediatrics, 101*(3 Pt 1), 486–489.

Davis, D. W., Jones, V. F., Logsdon, M. C., Ryan, L., & Wilkerson-McMahon, M. (2013). Health promotion in pediatric primary care: Importance of health literacy and communication practices. *Clinical Pediatrics (Phila), 52*(12), 1127–1134. doi:10.1177/0009922813506607.

Dunst, C. J., Johanson, C., Trivette, C. M., & Hamby, D. (1991). Family-oriented early intervention policies and practices: Family-centered or not? *Exceptional Children, 58*(2), 115–126.

Fazzone, P. A., Barloon, L. F., McConnell, S. J., & Chitty, J. A. (2000). Personal safety, violence, and home health. *Public Health Nursing, 17*(1), 43–52.

Goyal, N. K., Teeters, A., & Ammerman, R. T. (2013). Home visiting and outcomes of preterm infants: A systematic review. *Pediatrics, 132*(3), 502–516. doi:10.1542/peds.2013-0077.

Healthy Families America. (2014). *About us: Overview*. From http://www.healthyfamiliesamerica. org/about_us/index.shtml.

Holland, M. L., Christensen, J. J., Shone, L. P., Kearney, M. H., & Kitzman, H. J. (2014). Women's reasons for attrition from a nurse home visiting program. *Journal of Obstetric, Gynecologic, and Neonatal Nursing, 43*(1), 61–70. doi:10.1111/1552-6909.12263.

Issel, L. M., Forrestal, S. G., Slaughter, J., Wiencrot, A., & Handler, A. (2011). A review of prenatal home-visiting effectiveness for improving birth outcomes. *Journal of Obstetric, Gynecologic, and Neonatal Nursing, 40*(2), 157–165. doi:10.1111/j.1552-6909.2011.01219.x.

Love, J. M., Kisker, E. E., Ross, C., Raikes, H., Constantine, J., Boller, K., et al. (2005). The effectiveness of early head start for 3-year-old children and their parents: lessons for policy and programs. *Developmental Psychology, 41*(6), 885–901. doi:10.1037/0012-1649.41.6.88.

McCurdy, K. (2005). The influence of support and stress on maternal attitudes. *Child Abuse and Neglect, 29*(3), 251–268. doi:10.1016/j.chiabu.2004.12.007.

Nadwairski, J. A. (1992). Inner-city safety for home care providers. *Journal of Nursing Administration, 22*(9), 42–47.

National Healthy Start Association. (2014). Retrieved July 1, from http://www.national healthystart.org/

Nurse-Family Partnership. (2014). Retrieved July 1, from http://www.nursefamilypartnership.org/

O'Brien, R. A., Moritz, P., Luckey, D. W., McClatchey, M. W., Ingoldsby, E. M., & Olds, D. L. (2012). Mixed methods analysis of participant attrition in the nurse-family partnership. *Prevention Science, 13*(3), 219–228. doi:10.1007/s11121-012-0287-0.

Olds, D. (1992). Home visitation for pregnant women and parents of young children. *American Journal of Diseases of Children, 146*(6), 704–708.

Olds, D., Henderson, C. R, Jr, Kitzman, H., & Cole, R. (1995). Effects of prenatal and infancy nurse home visitation on surveillance of child maltreatment. *Pediatrics, 95*(3), 365–372.

Parents as Teachers. (2014). Retrieved 2014, from http://www.parentsasteachers.org/about.

Peacock, S., Konrad, S., Watson, E., Nickel, D., & Muhajarine, N. (2013). Effectiveness of home visiting programs on child outcomes: A systematic review. *BMC Public Health, 13*, 17. doi:10.1186/1471-2458-13-17.

Raikes, H., Green, B. L., Atwater, J., Kisker, E., Constantine, J., & Chazan-Cohen, R. (2006). Involvement in Early Head Start home visiting services: Demographic predictors and relations to child and parent outcomes. *Early childhood Research Quarterly, 21*, 2–24.

Smith, S. A., & Moore, E. J. (2012). Health literacy and depression in the context of home visitiation. *Maternal and Child Health Journal, 16*, 1500–1508.

Smithbattle, L., Lorenz, R., & Leander, S. (2013). Listening with care: Using narrative methods to cultivate nurses' responsive relationships in a home visiting intervention with teen mothers. *Nursing Inquiry, 20*(3), 188–198. doi:10.1111/j.1440-1800.2012.00606.x.

Strom, A., Kvernbekk, T., & Fagermoen, M. S. (2011). Parity: (im) possible? Interplay of knowledge forms in patient education. *Nursing Inquiry, 18*(2), 94–101. doi:10.1111/j.1440-1800.2011.00517.x.

U.S. Department of Health and Human Serivces. (2013). *Home visiting evidence of effectiveness*. Retrieved 2014, from http://homvee.acf.hhs.gov/Default.aspx.

Wagner, M., Spiker, D., & Linn, M. I. (2002). The effectiveness of the Parents as Teachers program with low-income parents and children. *TECSE, 22*(2), 67–81.

Wasik, B. H., Bryan, D. M., & Lyons, C. M. (1990). *Home visiting: procedures for helping families*. Newbury Park, California: Sage Publications.

Weiss, H. B. (1993). Home visits: Necessary but not sufficient. *Future of Children, 3*, 113–128.

Zeanah, P. D., Larrieu, J. A., Boris, N. W., & Nagle, G. (2006). Nurse home visiting: Perspecitives from nurses. *Infant Mental Health Journal, 27*, 41–54.

Chapter 8
Managed Care and Case Management

Children with special health care needs represent an important subgroup in managed care plans. Managed care plans focus on prevention/wellness programs and programs the support the highest level of function for individuals with congenital and/or chronic health conditions. At the disposal of the managed plans are units focused on relationships with providers, contracting, claims payment, and member services. The team focuses on addressing the needs of the individuals (termed members) that are served under the managed care plan. Specifically for children with special health care needs, the managed care is incented to help the family secure quality, organized, efficient services to avoid duplication, rework or dis-satisfaction. The federal Maternal and Child Health Bureau's Division of services for Children with Special Health Care Needs convened a work group to develop a definition that will give context to who this population is:

> Children with special health care needs are those who have or are at increased risk for a chronic physical, developmental, behavioral, or emotional condition and who also require health and related services of a type or amount beyond that required by children generally (U.S. Department of Health and Human Services, Health Resources and Services Administration 2007).

One of the benefits of managed care systems is their breadth of programming and emphasis on providing and measuring quality. Managed care plans have outreach programs for preventive care, chronic conditions and adolescent transition as well as programming addressing transition between care levels (Antonelli et al. 2009). Customer/family satisfaction ratings and fidelity to industry standards is also widely seen in plans as they seek to attain and maintain accreditation amidst their peers. Health care providers and well as families should be aware that certification exists as this is a mark of a wide availability of resources to families. Managed care companies obtain case management accreditation from national organizations and use that as a marketing tool as well as evidence of their level of performance. The movement into managed care of more individuals under the Affordable Care Act changes provides a new opportunity for children to receive

© The Author(s) 2015
J. Treadwell et al., *Case Management and Care Coordination*,
SpringerBriefs in Child Health, DOI 10.1007/978-3-319-07224-1_8

better coordination of care and for data to be available to substantiate the provision of the highest standards of case management.

Tips for Families: Ask if your managed care case management program is URAC Accredited or NCQA Certified. This means that the organization meets national best practices in case management and promotes quality including offering patients and their caregivers' information on their programs and information on Consumer rights and responsibilities will be provided to you.

Tips for Health Care Professionals: Managed care organizations have robust case management programs. Connect your patients to the program through a referral back to the managed care plan.

Managed Care has a variety of structuring and reimbursement tools for health care. Many of those include holding providers accountable for providing a certain level of quality care based on measures with national benchmarks. Response time to family calls, the time it takes to pay a claim, use of physician-developed guidelines for addressing chronic illness are all components of this quality infra-structure. There are many different types of managed care plans. There are both Medicaid, Medicare and employee based managed care plans (also called Commercial plans). Individuals can belong to one or more of these plan types depending on their qualification. For example a child may qualify for commercial coverage under a parent's insurance coverage and also have Medicaid insurance coverage from another managed care plan for services not covered by the parent's policy. In managed care plans, children/members chose a primary care provider from a network of providers. This site of care is referred to as the medical home and can be an important decision as your child's primary care provider and specialists need to be within the contracted network of your chosen managed care plan. It is important to make sure the pediatric provider is within the contracted network of your managed care plan and that they agree to provide services for children with special needs. Many children's hospital systems offer a health plan or there are special pediatric networks that have affiliated with select managed care plans to deliver the array of services a child with special needs may require.

Some parents may elect to have both parents obtain insurance coverage to maxi-mize benefits. This is another way in which a child may have a care relationship with more than one managed care plan. Expensive medications are often covered under a pharmacy benefit of the health plan and other types of home care services are covered under the medical benefit with vision and dental care provided under still other benefits (Table 8.1). Some managed care plans require all care be conducted within a specific network while others allow children to use out-of-network provider at a higher share of cost. Researching the provisions prior to seeking care is essential and involves the health care provider and the family. The health plan case manager can assist in guiding services to locations which will be less of a financial burden to the family.

Managed care is a comprehensive approach to providing and paying for high quality health care services from educational resources and emergency services to complex inpatient care, all in a cost effective and coordinated system. The most common of managed care plan type are Health Maintenance Organizations

Table 8.1 Basic benefits that may be covered or provided by managed care plans

Healthcare
    Medical
    Dental
    Psychiatric
    Dental
    Vision
    Audiology
    Prescription drugs
    Substance abuse
    Nutritionist
    Specialty drug therapy
    Orthotics and prosthetics
    Preventative health care and screening

Therapy
    Physical
    Occupational
    Speech
    Respiratory

Psychology

Skilled nursing

Durable medical equipment
    Wheelchairs
    Hospital beds
    Walker
    Respiratory equipment including oxygen

*Other disability services that may be provided in the community and not under the managed
care health plan*

Special education services in schools

Assistive technologies and devices
    Devices for the visually impaired
    Devices for the hearing impaired
    Hardware/software systems

Personal assistance and supervision
    In-residence care
    Meal preparation and feeding
    Housekeeping and laundry
    Shopping
    Transportation to appointments
    Cognitive impairment supervision

Home Modification and environmental controls
    Wide doors and ramps

(continued)

Table 8.1 (continued)

Air quality control
Family respite care
Community programs
Recreation
Transportation
Adult day care
Training
Skills for the visually impaired
Skills for the hearing impaired
Life skills
Employment and vocational skills
Residential services
Vehicle modifications
Wheelchair loading

Centers for Medicare and Medicaid Services (2013)

(HMOs). Preferred Provider Organizations (PPO's) are another managed care option available in the Commercial (employer-based) population. If there are options to choose a plan, it is important to do some research prior to selection. The American Academy of Pediatrics has been a leader in helping parents learn to use their managed care plan effectively and has supported early intervention by linking services for children with special needs. Their website, aap.org, can be of great help when determining attributes of a managed care plan to select, as well as in setting expectations for services.

Medicaid is a government program that provides medical assistance for qualified beneficiaries. Most states offer an array of managed care options for Medicaid eligible children with special needs to receive their health care from networks developed by managed care organizations (Hughes et al. 1995). Families of Medicaid-eligible children with special care needs and/or disabilities must make a selection of managed care plans based on the network and benefits provided. If the parent/guardian does not select a primary care provider when they select a plan, the health plan will assign one. Once enrolled the child receives an identification card, a member handbook, provider directory and information on the process called prior authorization.

There is an advantage in having a case manager assigned to a child. The Health Maintenance Organization (HMO) or Preferred Provider Organization (PPO) typically has a process in place to automatically assign a for outreach once they have reviewed claim history and found a pattern of services or a specific diagnosis that triggers an alert for extra service.

Tips for Family: Make sure when enrolling a child in a managed care plan, to identify if case management services are automatic or by request. In most health plans, the guardian of a child can request case management services and skip the delay of waiting until the claims history indicates a need.

Health care providers participating in the managed care network can also initiate case management through a referral. Physicians and facilities partner with the managed care plan to help identify children/families needing support in coordinating care. The assigned case manager is typically a registered nurse or social worker. The child's case manager works with the parent/caregiver and the child as well as providers to develop an individual health care plan based on a health assessment, and goals. The case manager knows what is available in the managed care network, giving the family information on how to most effectively access services needed. The case manager monitors services even those provided outside the HMO or PPO. The managed care case manager acts as an advocate for the child, recommending services outside the network when access is not possible inside of contracted providers. An advantage of the case manager in managed care plans, is the provision of continuity across in and out of network care resulting in better coordination of services to meet the child's needs.

Case management programs in managed care plans are designed to provide support to children with special needs and their families, while linking them to resources and services in their own communities (Wise et al., 2007). Case managers are professionally prepared individuals and often act as a mediator between family and the service delivery system as they perform individual service planning, service coordination and monitoring as they understand available benefits of the plan as well as clinical and social needs of the child/family.

Many managed care plans offer field case management. It is important to identify if field case management is a benefit of the benefit plan of the child with special needs. This is especially important if the child has ongoing medical or therapy services. The field case manager comes to the home and helps evaluate what is needed and satisfaction with the network providers delivering care. They can also meet the child/family at the doctor's office or therapist appointment to assist in coordination of care and referrals that may be needed.

8.1 Important Components of Managed Care Case Management for Families

A case manager's role is defined by the amount of support and interventions a child/family needs. Services can range from intensive to informational. Parents are given the option to verbally consent to be in a case management program. A welcome packet is usually sent to the parent outlining their rights and responsibilities.

What you can expect from Case Management Program in Managed Care

• Providing Information
  The case manager will provide the family and child with information regarding the child's diagnosis, information to support shared-decision making, listings of support groups, applicable resources, and services from which the child and family may benefit.

- Connecting a Child to Needed Services
  The case manager facilitates access to network services to meet their children's needs such as physical therapy, occupational and speech therapy. The case manager can also act as an advocate for needs to be met through the school and individualized education plan, or identify services outside of the contracted network. Many case managers can authorize field case management home care visits and attendants when warranted for children with disabling conditions.
- Assisting with Transition
  The case manager assists a child and family with transitioning from in-patient to home setting. Coordinating with multiple providers can help a family when they need services most and help them prioritize care. Explaining benefit provisions and limitations supports the child/family in choices for arranging care.
- Special Disease Management Programs
  Managed care plans offer disease management programs for specific populations with chronic illnesses like sickle cell disease, complex congenital heart disease, juvenile diabetes, genetic syndromes, or multiple complications of extreme prematurity. These ongoing programs are dedicated to look at use of benefits and services to deliver improved outcomes. Case managers with advanced training are utilized in these special programs. They can help a family plan for changes in care needs and use reminder systems to support adherence to treatment plans.
- Patient Centered Medical Home Programs
  Many managed care plans are promoting their pediatric and family practice provider networks to obtain Patient Centered Medical Home Achievement or Certification from a national accreditation body such as URAC, The Joint Commission, or the National Commission for Quality Assurance. There is often a close working relationship with the case manager from the managed care health plan and the Patient Centered Medical Home. This additional network requirement identifies to consumers, practices willing to embrace a patient centered focus on care coordination. Case managers or community outreach staff can help families select a pediatrician that has this special designation.

8.2 What are the Specific Duties and Responsibilities of the Managed Care Case Manager?

The managed care case manager works with both children and their parents. In a family-centered approach, the case manager families leads through the maze of the health service system and other related systems and are responsible for providing many of the following services:

   I. Intake Assessment and individualized care plan.
  II. Counseling on benefit plan provisions, care choices, and programs available in the managed care plan that supply services applicable to the child. Being available to the families as a resource in a crisis, responding actively to complaints about services and providing objective information about alternatives for securing direct services.
 III. Facilitation of communication among multiple providers servicing families including the primary health care provider.
 IV. Monitoring services received by families by reviewing the child's progress toward the attainment of prioritized goals identified in the individual care plan.

8.3 Learning to Partner with Your Case Manager

The relationship between healthcare professionals, families and the case manager is one of a team. Looking at this relationship as a partnership, communication is important. Organizing medical and managed care reports and papers into files can help all parties (Table 8.2). Understanding the case manager is advocating for the optimal health interests of the child helps establish necessary trust during the stresses of caregiving and parenting the special needs child (Table 8.3). Managed care case managers suggest families will want to keep:

- A journal to write down questions for the care team and concerns
- A plan of care and emergency protocol
- Medication lists
- Physician's orders
- Reports from Specialists and/or Therapists
- Lab and test results
- Evaluations
- Records of home visits and home agency's nursing care plan
- Nutritional plans
- Daily routines
- Important phone numbers (including that of the case manager) and,
- Insurance information

Case managers working in managed care plan can also link children to additional state waiver programs. The case managers understand qualifying conditions and facilitate enrollment of wait-listing for these additional benefits and/or other resources to help in advocating for a child's healthcare needs (Table 8.4). These waiver programs were designed for highly specialized populations such as developmentally disabled beneficiaries and need to be evaluated for coordination or replacement of other insurance coverage. Ask your case manager about qualifications or check your state Medicaid web site or call their department for special needs children services. Optional benefits which may be covered by states include:

Table 8.2 How to create a detailed file for your special needs child

Patient file (paper or electronic)
Being prepared for an emergency or a visit to a new provider makes sense. Caregivers can create and maintain a comprehensive file of information about the child support comprehensive communication exchange. There are a variety of ways to create and maintain a healthcare file. Paper, or electronic, the idea is to have quick access to a summary of the child's history and present treatment/condition. Check to see if your managed care plan offers a PHR (patient health record) electronically online for you to access. The PHR allows you to add your own information as well as have access to claim and provider information about your child
If you choose a paper format, store in a place you will remember in an emergency
Keep it up to date after any changes in medications treatments, or procedures
Include:

Medical History
        Diagnosis, allergies
        Physician contact information
        Treatment history (e.g. surgeries, other medical conditions)

Medication listing (including dosing and frequency)
Insurance information   Medical insurance cards, ID, policy

Legal documents
        Living will
        Durable power of attorney for Health Care (also known as a Health Care Proxy)
        Contact information for child's lawyer if applicable

Table 8.3 Top 5 mistakes for parents to avoid

1	*Not being pro-active.* Parents must be the ones to make things happen for their children! To do this effectively, they must arm themselves with information about insurance, health benefits as well as what treatment options are available. A can-do attitude will be contagious to their child who needs to be the best they can be. They also need to know more about children's disabilities and legal rights. Find a case manager that has expertise in coordinating services that will partner with the parent
2	*Not keeping important papers in one place.* Parents cannot remember everything without an organized system to find important health records and insurance information when they need it. Being organized will help to access services
3	*Not networking with other parents of special needs children.* Parents cannot afford to be isolated and support groups can offer valuable help. Isolations lead to stress and being overwhelmed. Take time to network on line or in person to support groups and connect with other parents
4	*Ruining your relationships with health care providers and school staff.* Parents who argue and are rude will not get heard. Parents are more likely to receive cooperation from staff if they maintain amicable relations with them. It is okay to be assertive when asking for supports for your children but avoid being argumentative
5	*Failing to research and choose a primary care physician that offers medical home services.* Parents may be very frustrated with primary care providers that have very little experience with special needs children. Parents need to do some research to see if the provider network in the managed care plan has family practice or pediatric providers that offer medical home services with nutrition, case management and preventative health services. Be prepared to ask questions about services offered to special needs children and parents before you choose a doctor

Table 8.4 Helpful links

CMS Centers for Medicare and Medicaid Services
Website http://cms.hhs.gov
A federal Web site to helping you learn more about services and Medicaid benefits

U.S. Department of Health and Human Services
Website www.healthfinder.gov
A federal Web site designed to help people stay healthy. Healthfinder.gov features links to more than 6,000 government and nonprofit health information resources on hundreds of health topics including personalized health tools such as health calculators, activity and menu planners, recipes, and online checkups. In addition, the site offers tips for caregivers and health news. Information is provided in both English and Spanish

CareConnection.com
Website http://www.careconnection.com
CareConnection.com is a Website devoted to family caregivers, with up-to-date health news, elder care specialists, experts, insurance help, and coping advice. The site, owned by HealthCentral.com, offers in-depth resources from trusted sources, interactive tools, and connections to leading experts and caregivers who share their experiences and inspiration.

Disability.gov
Website http://www.disability.gov/
A federal government website providing easy access to disability-related information and resources, Disability.gov has links to relevant programs and services offered by numerous government agencies. It is designed as a one-stop website where people with disabilities can easily find the resources they need to fully participate in the workforce and in their communities. Included is a state and local resources map, which makes it easy to locate disability-related information in specific parts of the country

National Institutes of Health (NIH)
Find information on health topics and disability
http://www.nih.gov

Family Voices, Inc.
888-835-5669
Website http://www.familyvoices.org
Family voices offers information on healthcare policies relevant to special needs children in every state

Medicine Program
573-996-7300
Website http://www.themedicineprogram.com
This program is for persons who do not have coverage either through insurance or government subsidies for outpatient prescription drugs and for those who cannot afford to purchase medications at retail prices

Patient Advocate Foundation
800-532-5274
Patient Advocate Foundation serves as a liaison between patients and their insurer, employer and/or creditors to resolve insurance, job retention and/or debt crisis matters relating to a patient's condition
www.patientadvocate.org

Visiting Nurse Associations of America
617-737-3200
Website http://www.vnaa.org
e-mail: vnaa@vnaa.org

(continued)

Table 8.4 (continued)

VNAA promotes community based home healthcare. Family caregivers can contact them to find their local VNA
Easter Seals 800-221-6827 *Website* http://www.easter-seals.org Toll-free: 800-233-4050 *Website* http://www.chadd.org Easter Seals provides a variety of services at 400 sites nationwide for children and adults with disabilities, including adult day care, in-home care, camps for special needs children and more. Services vary by site
National Alliance on Mental Illness *Website* www.nami.org This site offers up to date information on Medicaid Expansion Programs in different states and news on the Accountable Care Act and exchange health plans
Healthy Children *Website* www.healthychildren.org This site has information on managed care plans and how to get good care for your child

- Medical or remedial care
- Immediate care facility services for individuals under the age of 21
- Personal care services
- Private duty nursing services
- Respiratory care for vent—dependent individuals
- Home and community based services
- Services for individuals with speech, hearing and language impairments

Managed care case managers are educated to be involved with parents to help them prepare for every stage of their child's life through special needs life care planning. There are key stages of special needs planning associated with age and/ or developmental needs of the child. In life care planning the future needs of the child is considered along with the findings of treating providers and specialists. The developmental age of the child is an important consideration not just the chronological age of the child. Gaps in care are identified so planning is done to accommodate these issues. For instance a child with cerebral palsy may require different types of adaptive devices and upgrades to motorized wheelchairs as they get older and access to physical therapists and occupational therapists that do proper fittings for wheelchairs. Some benefit provisions limit the frequency of equipment purchase so planning is important. These plans need to be coordinated with the ordering provider. In life care planning it is critical to look at what insurance will pay for and share with the primary care or specialist provider how often replacements and upgrades of equipment are allowed. Access to financial planning is also part of a comprehensive life care plan for a child with special needs. Life care planning was created to help integrate resources, legal planning and health care needs to ensure a brighter future for a person with a disability. Most states have focused on children under 17 and often long range planning is needed to look at comprehensive services. Parents in Dealing with Managed Care Plans

Maintaining important records or documents in one place is a good strategy. These important records or documents include the child's health policy and identification numbers, your child's health plan ID card, telephone numbers of contact people, copies of all letters from the managed care plan, doctors, case managers, etc. notes from all visits and services had by your child.

> Tips for families: When you talk to someone at the managed care plan write down the date, time and the person's name. If something they say seems important, ask them to put it in writing and send it to you. Keep these records. Try to get the number of the same customer service representative so when you call for information on coverage and benefits they know you.

Families should be encouraged to talk to their primary care provider on what kinds of services may be needed and if their insurance coverage has restrictions in the amount or cost allowed. The case manager may be required to request a benefit exception to allow non-covered services. The managed care case manager can guide the team in explaining how exceptions are made in the organization. The case manager will reinforce the importance of building a strong and positive relationship with their medical home. For commercial managed care plans, be sure to keep the name of the benefits manager in charge of health benefits at your work or a benefits manager/case management supervisor within the Medicaid managed care plan as well as the toll free hotline or ombudsman program in your state. Another area where a case manager can assist is in the area of prescription medication. It is important for financial responsibility of the family to be mitigated through use of formulary medications. The case manager can have discussion with the prescribing providers to discuss medications which are on formulary or where generic medications are available. The case manager can also help families in submitting for mail-order prescriptions to obtain a more reasonable price. Some medications must be obtained at specialty or compounding pharmacies, the case manager can explain what pharmacies are part of the managed care network and how processing and ordering may be most efficiently achieved. If there is a need to speak to your managed care plan about claims, attempt to speak with the same claims supervisor or your case manager. Ask for the name and phone number of the representative and try to speak with that person every time. This will help you from having to repeat your child's story. Similarly, when obtaining authorizations for therapy, equipment or prescriptions from your managed care plan contact your case manager to understand the procedure regarding prior authorization. Your managed care plan may require a letter of medical necessity, or the written prescription forms from your primary care physician, which the case manager can help you obtain.

If you receive a claim denial, it will be in writing. It should include the specific reason for the denial. Managed care companies are legally obligated to provide this. Families and providers may question denials, and if you believe the claim is valid, appeal the denial and resubmit the claim. Be sure to sign release of information so all the records will be released to support your claim. Managed care health plans are regulated by state government. To report issues, contact your State Insurance Commission. State governments require a response from the managed care plan in a certain time frame and they can expedite an appeal.

It is important to remember that for school age children with special health care needs the school system is also responsible to offer services. The passage of the Individuals with Disabilities Education Act (Idea 97) created provisions to give parents of children with special needs the legal means to ensure their children's needs are met at school. Individualized education plans (IEP's) and 504 plans are two options to carefully investigate as your child nears the school—age years. Parents who engage with a health plan case manager can sign a release of information so the Health Plan Case manager participates in review these plans. The case manager can be an advocate in situations such as when a child with physical disabilities needs extra time during school meals yet the school has not addressed this issue. In some cases a field case manager can go into the school to check that the IEP and 504 plans are being implemented (Mullahy 2014).

In conclusion, case management in managed care has helped find solutions that support children and families. Case managers who work with special needs children in managed care programs offer expertise in health care and community services in addition to understanding how to navigate through managed care requirements of authorizations, benefits, and appeals. Case managers enable consumers to obtain the best value for their insurance in maximizing the wellness of their child.

References

Antonelli, R., McAllister, J., & Popp, J. (2009). Managing care coordination a critical component of the pediatric health system: a multidisciplinary framework. *The Commonwealth Fund.* Retrieved from http://www.commonwealthfund.org/~/media/Files/Publications/Fund%20 Report/2009/May/Making%20Care%20Coordination%20a%20Critical%20Component/ 1277_Antonelli_making_care_coordination_critical_FINAL.pdf.

Centers for Medicare and Medicaid Services. (2013). Chapter 4—benefits and beneficiary protections. *Medicare managed care manual.* Retrieved from http://www.cms.gov/ Regulations-and-Guidance/Guidance/Manuals/downloads/mc86c04.pdf.

Hughes, D., Newacheck, P., Stoddard, J., & Halfon, N. (1995). Medicaid managed care: Can it work for children? *Pediatrics.* Retrieved from http://pediatrics.aappublications.org/content/ 95/4/591.full.pdf+html.

Mullahy, C. (2014). *The case manager's handbook.* Boston: Jones and Bartlett Learning.

U.S. Department of Health and Human Services, Health Resources and Services Administration, Maternal and Child Health Bureau. (2007). *The National Survey of Children with Special Health Care Needs Chartbook 2005–2006.* Rockville, Maryland: U.S. Department of Health and Human Services.

Wise, P., Huffman, L., & Brat, G. (2007, June). AHRQ Publication No. 07-0054 A Critical Analysis of Care Coordination Strategies for Children with Special Health Care Needs. AHRQ Publication No. 07-0054. Retrieved from http://www.ncbi.nlm.nih.gov/books/NBK44054/.

Wright, H. (2013). *The complete guide to creating a special needs life plan*. Philadelphia: Jessica Kingsley Publishers.

Chapter 9
Technology

9.1 Explanation of Technology Impacting Care Coordination

The Affordable Care Act is influencing the use of technology in areas of quality healthcare, health services delivery, and patient engagement. Health information technology references come in an array of acronyms. It is useful to untangle these terms and definitions as technology provide a significant benefit to families and children in accessing information and services as well as in improving quality (Table 9.1). Health information technology (you will see referred to as HIT) has the foundational element of combining information about an individual (child) from various sources so the health care professional delivering care has an integrated and actionable view of health history and health status. Within a hospital setting or even within connected clinics this is not too difficult if a child frequents the same set of providers. However, across different hospitals and delivering physicians, therapy companies, or supply vendors, the creation of a health record electronically depends on a health information exchange (HIE). Acceptance of use of HIE technology is occurring but definitely not on a universal basis. Integration of health care information at a comprehensive level is facilitated in part by what is known as "Stage 2 of Meaningful Use." Effective January 2014 health care professionals must use HIT to optimize care coordination (Teich 2013). The Federal government first gave hospitals and physicians support funding to pay for equipment and training to implement electronic records and to receive continued financial subsidy they must now use the technology for the purpose of care coordination. These financial incentives are propelling adoption of electronic records and HIE adoption across the United States. This is a great thing for both families and health care providers as establishing health information exchanges and developing technology infrastructure improves quality, reduce costs; and improves care coordination across hospitals, labs, pharmacies, physicians and other all types of delivery entities while ensuring security of information (Fig. 9.1).

© The Author(s) 2015
J. Treadwell et al., *Case Management and Care Coordination*,
SpringerBriefs in Child Health, DOI 10.1007/978-3-319-07224-1_9

Table 9.1 Definition of Health Information Technology Terms

The National Alliance for Health Information Technology (NAHIT) was assigned to develop national definitions for the terms EMR, EHR, PHR, HIE, HIO, and RHIO resulting in adoption of the following definitions:

Electronic Medical Record (EMR)—An electronic record of health-related information on an individual that can be created, gathered, managed, and consulted by authorized clinicians and staff within one health care organization

Electronic Health Record (EHR)—An electronic record of health-related information on an individual that conforms to nationally recognized interoperability standards and that can be created, managed, and consulted by authorized clinicians and staff across more than one health care organization

Personal Health Record (PHR)—An electronic record of health-related information on an individual that conforms to nationally recognized interoperability standards and that can be drawn from multiple sources while being managed, shared, and controlled by the individual

Health Information Exchange (HIE)—The electronic movement of health-related information among organizations according to nationally recognized standards (verb)

Health Information Organization (HIO)—An organization that oversees and governs the exchange of health-related information among organizations according to nationally recognized standards (noun)

Regional Health Information Organization (RHIO)—A health information organization that brings together health care stakeholders within a defined geographic area and governs health information exchange among them for the purpose of improving health and care in that community

Adapted from http://www.nacua.org/documents/HealthInfoTechTerms.pdf. The National Alliance for Health Information Technology, 2008

> Tips for Parents: Be prepared to answer the question of your preference to consent to your child's health information shared across providers. Understand that access to a complete picture of your child's health may reduce duplication, errors, and your need to repeat a lengthy medical history yet again.
>
> Tip for Health Care Professional: Signing onto an HIE is one step in providing consistent care for your patients.

Although helpful in communication, primary care offices have adopted use of many different kinds of electronic health systems (EHR) which sets up barriers for easy information transfer. The Office of the National Coordinator for Health Information Technology (ONC), is a position legislated in the HITECH Act, that is charged with improving connection of health information technology infrastructure and development on a national level. One area of development is that of a personal health record (PHR). A PHR aggregates information such as allergies, immunizations, family history, medications, hospital records, and records of office visits into one file that contains a full picture of an individual (child's) health. However, consent to allow your child's health information to be shared across providers must be gained by the child's legally authorized representative.

So how does this help coordinate a child's care most effectively? One example can be seen in the instance a child has both physical health and behavioral health needs to address. In this situation, it is important that each discipline be aware of the medications and testing result of the child to make sure no untoward

Fig. 9.1 Information Health
Network. *Source* healthit.gov

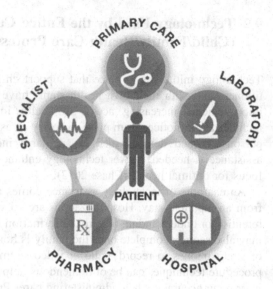

interaction occurs and each practitioner understand necessary laboratory monitoring involved in care. Another example of HIE advantage would be if a child was
visiting outside a reasonable transportation range of their medical home and
needed to seek services at an emergency center. Having access to past medical
records, including an accurate listing of current medications and treatment, would
avoid duplication of testing and allow the provider to understand what normal
thresholds of function exist for this specific child, something that could easily
prevent duplication of testing and a more efficient focus on the acute reason the
child presented for treatment. If a part of the treatment required radiography, the
wait for a physician to read the films would be decreased as the 'picture' could be
transmitted to any location for a radiologist review, speeding the diagnosis and
move to appropriate treatment.

Treatment of children with multiple and/or chronic conditions demonstrates
optimal use of this technology sharing as each specialty has a part to play in
supporting maximum function and outcomes (Antonelli, 2013). Providing a view
where every person can understand what the other has ordered or planned, assists
in setting goals and measuring progress along the course of treatment. Tracking of
laboratory values, such as the blood sugar levels in children with diabetes, helps in
family management of the child's day to day care, delivering consistent information to both caregivers and care providers. Engagement and shared decision
making is enhanced with use of the clinical information. The data created in the
PHR can also be evaluated, using sophisticated analytics to predict next steps and
response to evidenced based guidelines.

9.2 Technology Used by the Entire Care Team (Child/Family/Health Care Professionals)

Technology initiatives in place that support child/family engagement with practitioners and with their own health status have been enhanced through internet improvements increasing access to health information. Familiar technology includes alarm notices from pulse oximetry or assistive respiratory equipment and person-activated devices such as an alarm indicating a child has fallen and assistance is needed. Newer technology enhances engagement which is a major focus for optimal health (Chase 2012).

An example of technology assistance comes at the time of a child's discharge from an inpatient stay. Hospitalizations are so stressful for the entire family that retention or understanding of verbal information is limited and written information may also seem incomplete once the family is home and caring for their child. Use of smart phones to record audio or video segments of discharge instructions or procedure techniques can be of tremendous help to families in reducing stress and improving accuracy when administering care. Prior to discharge, as a component of care coordination, information is being shared more freely during patient stays to improve understanding of medications and treatments. An example, Main Line Health in Pennsylvania has developed a Patient Daily Care Plan from electronic patient record information (Glaser 2013). This printout familiarizes families with medications, specialists names, pending studies as well as current treatments. The National Transitions of Care Coalition has published a white paper defining necessary technology elements of care transition which include strong care coordination and use of goals to engage accountability (Stricker 2013).

Reminder technology, expanding from automated reminder phone calls, has spread to text reminders for appointments as well as the need to complete testing prior to a health care appointment. Scheduling, as well, can be completed online for many primary care and specialty practices including calendar reminders automatically being sent to families to improve successful attendance. Once in the office setting, a tablet device or health kiosk is an increasingly accepted way to update demographic information as well as complete survey instruments on a child's development. These entries are automatically scored so the primary care provider can incorporate the results in the visit within minutes, reducing the need for a second visit (http://www.pedstest.com/OnlineScreening.aspx).

If chronic health conditions or developmental delays are identified, technology can be employed in ongoing monitoring, development of an online care plan, and interaction in health coaching, and case management delivery. Ongoing monitoring opportunities vary according to health need including such items as biometric monitoring of blood glucose, pulmonary function, weight which transmit information to treating practitioners and include an alert feature for instances when values are outside of set parameters. These devices require child/family engagement as well as integration with a healthcare provider.

Table 9.2 Care Plan Components

Health	Visual and hearing needs/preferences limitations
Consent	Caregiver resources and involvement
Strengths and needs assessment	Early childhood intervention services
Community resources	Prioritized goals
Condition specific issues	Barriers to meeting goals
Clinical history	Referrals to resources and follow up to determine success of link
Assessment of activities of daily living	Scheduled communication plan
Mental health status assessment	Self management plan
Cultural and linguistic needs/preferences/limitations	Life planning

One of most important supports to care coordination is the care plan. The care plan is a comprehensive document that gives a picture of the past and present child's health status, prioritized needs and preferences in a context of patient history and planned treatments/care. Included are items such as current medications, names of all care providers, and recent test results (Table 9.2). The optimal case plan is online so that the patient/family, medical home practitioner, specialists, and ancillary providers may all see the common thread supporting a consistent plan of care. For example, a daily blood sugar can be logged or exercise activity alongside clinical values such as a HA1c or LDL level. Family entries and practitioner entries develop into a more robust picture of need and achievements supporting optimal outcomes for the child. The interactive plan of care is an important part of the Patient Health Record (PHR), which will be discussed in the next section.

Another valuable technological tool shared by the patient/family and care providers is telemedicine. Telemedicine is being used more and more, validating technology assisted care can be successful in improving capacity for certain provider types which may have low availability due to specialization or geography. An example would be child psychiatrists or neurologists, who are in high demand due to low numbers of these practicing professionals.

These physicians tend to practice in metropolitan and often academic settings. Using alternative sites for service, such as a primary care office, the child/family can connect to the provider through a secure internet portal and engage in needed services while supported in the care location by ancillary healthcare staff. This mode of delivery enhances the capacity of physical and behavioral health treatment for families who would otherwise lack service.

Care providers as well as patients and families can additionally use technology to access quality standards of treatment specific to health conditions. Access to practice guidelines, developed through research and professional consensus enables parents to set realistic expectations of the type and amount of services. The most notable of sources for pediatric guidelines include:

American   Academy   of   Pediatrics   http://pediatrics.aappublications.org/site/
aappolicy/
American Academy of Child and Adolescent Psychiatry http://www.aacap.org/
AACAP/Resources_for_Primary_Care/Practice_Parameters_and_Resource_Centers/
Practice_Parameters.aspx
National Guideline Clearinghouse http://www.guideline.gov/

> Tips for Parents: Ask your child's health care provider what guidelines they are following.
> Ask your provider or case manager for a copy or web site address. Understand that access
> to a complete picture of your child's health may reduce duplication, errors, and your need
> to repeat a lengthy medical history yet again.

> Tip for Health Care Professional: Sharing expectations with families supports their
> engagement and compliance in your evidenced based treatment plan.

9.3 Technology for Children/Families

Patient portals, are sites that allow access to the patient health record (PHR) and
also provide educational healthcare content specific to the child's demogrpahics.
Many insurance carriers host these portals for the benefit of care coordination
across their covered population (Roper et al. 2013). An example of a portal use has
been developed by the Verizon Foundation, in association with Johns Hopkins
University, UCLA, Harvard University and Emory University. They have developed a disease-management program using a wireless biometric device (glucom-
eter, scale) to integrate with an online portal that can be accessed remotely by the
child/family from any smart device or computer. The goal is to improve
engagement through easy access to health information, and individualized
treatment plan, and provider communication (http://responsibility.verizon.com/
healthcare/breaking-down-barriers-to-chronic-disease-care).

The portal is also a good entryway to links on information about your child's
diagnosis or links to providers in your area that participate in your child's health
plan. An advantage of researching diagnosis and treatment information through the
portal is the screening the portal does to make sure you are receiving information
from a site that is accurate in the information they share. Random searches on the
internet may lead the reader in the wrong direction if they come from entities that
are marketing a treatment or they may represent information without an evidence
basis. Shared decision making is a goal of information research, so it is important
to communicate your information and the sites that have been beneficial to you
with your care coordination team and health care providers. Pediatric sites may
also offer the option of individualized pages where the child or adolescent might
enter their likes and dislikes, such as they like to read, love NASCAR racing and
like to be called by a nickname. This information helps the team in communication
and understanding of the child an improving the trust relationship vital in care
coordination. Knowing the child/family's desires and preferences improves

engagement and treatment plan follow through because the child/family have a say in the process and the plan is tailored specifically toward them.

Expanding on that idea of children expression through a web page if the ability for a more expanded site hosted among a group of peers. Caring Bridges, a site that lets families develop secure sites that allow information to be shared and encouraging messages left (http://www.caringbridge.org/) is an example of a place where children can build their own pages and also converse with other children of like condition. Support systems to the family can also use the calendar page to organize information like when to bring meals on days of special treatments or arranging rides for the family. This type of technology can provide peer support to children who may be isolated from typical school interaction due to frequently missed school days or homebound status. Good examples for you to link to include: Kids Health (powered by Nemours) http://kidshealth.org/ and BraveKids (powered by United Cerebral Palsy) http://www.bravekids.org/.

Online support groups can be a benefit to parents as well. Addressing the barriers of work schedules and geography, online support groups can assist families in realistic expectations and most importantly get tips from people who have been experiencing a very similar reality. Creative ideas abound that don't have to be reinvented as families share what works and what does not work in terms of practices of caring for a child with special health care needs. One examples of such resources are: When your child is diagnosed with a chronic condition: how to cope, American Psychological Association found at http://www.apa.org/helpcenter/chronic-illness-child.aspx. Autism Speaks, an organization of education, support and advocacy relating to autism, has online parent support groups (http://www.autismspeaks.org/community-and-support-network/online-support-groups) as do groups associated with many other conditions. Siblings of children with special health care conditions can also benefit from technology and link to support groups. An example of one such resource a family can explore is Sibling Support http://www.siblingsupport.org/.

Families need to know what State programs exist that provide services or advocacy for children with special healthcare needs. Each State varies in program offerings. You can find information on the resources available in your State by linking to State Title V/Children with Special Healthcare Needs contact (select your State) https://mchdata.hrsa.gov/TVISReports/ContactInfo/StateContactSearch.aspx.

Noting that communication is key, use of the care coordination team to improve that communication can occur with technology. Many programs offer free IPads to children with communication delays or the child may receive a more sophisticated language board through their school system. Often a case manager can be of assistance to the family in advocating for such equipment from state agencies or school districts. Free educational applications are available for the technology that increase the child's success in communicating, a tremendous benefit for the child in expressing their desires and acquiring new skills.

Maintaining a link to the medical home and care coordinator is a fundamental use of technology using texting or emails. Texting has become a preferred method for many individuals due to the proliferation of Smartphones. Smartphones can be used for texting or emailing providers a question about a treatment or a change in symptoms, in some cases decreasing the need for transportation to a face-to-face appointment. Interaction with the care coordination team conducted through email erases any barriers of asking a questions during specific hours which can speed response time. Additionally, many families use smartphone applications (apps) to research quick information about healthcare topics such as medications or researching provider locations or experience. More than 17,000 healthcare smartphone apps were available as of September 2013 with the number growing daily (Frie 2013).

> Tips for Parents: Ask your child's health care provider and case manager/care coordination team member how you can utilize texting or emails to exchange information. Remember to ask about their policy on response time

> Tip for Health Care Professional: Depending on the child's insurance coverage, online interaction with the family may be reimbursable. Investigate the payment options for time you devote to your patients using technology assistance.

9.4 Technology Employed by Health Professionals

An example of a technology helpful in identifying individuals who could benefit from care coordination is predictive modeling applications. History of the child's use of health services (use of medical claims) combined with their age, gender, medication refill patterns and even zip code is analyzed by a highly developed set of algorithms which predict the likelihood of an emergency room visit or a service cost in the next 3 or 12 months. The modeling uses decision trees based upon sets of information from around the country on children of like age, diagnoses, and patterns of health use. Case managers use this information for identification and then, in concert with feedback loops in the system applications, can measure profession financial and clinical metrics. This same technology supports disease registries of individuals with like conditions and care cap modeling identifying individuals who are missing some vital testing or visits requirements as compared to best practice treatments for their condition.

Technology registries related to care coordination are beneficial at a practice level and are also useful at an organizational and State/National level. Group practices and integrated delivery systems of providers used combined registries for patient outreach and pay-for—performance/risk bearing strategies. On a state and national level computerized registries have existed for quite some time for identification of individuals immunization, type and stage of cancer or reportable communicable disease. Now registries exist at both the state and organizational levels inclusive of people with high risk deliveries, frequent emergency room utilization or admission/readmission rates.

There is general acceptance that children with special healthcare needs benefit from a medical home. Technology support to develop medical homes is available from the American Academy of Pediatrics and Center for Medical Home Improvement toolkit. The organizations have developed an online toolkit which can be individually modified by a practitioner to support development or improvement of medical homes (http://www.pediatricmedhome.org). This is important in the provision of quality, individualized care to patients as well as in effort to achieve accreditation from the National Committee for Quality Assurance (NCQA). The accredited medical home is increasingly becoming a requirement for participation in or improved payment levels in managed care networks. This medical home model is founded in care coordination and gains strength from the care plan based upon child/family involvements and shared decision-making.

Electronic receipt of test results, for example laboratory results has been in place for quite some time supporting care coordination through follow up with patients and assessment and communication of next steps of care based on test findings. Newer technology has expanded that concept into computerized decision support systems (CDSS). Care coordination can be enhanced through CDSS reminders for guideline adherence in children with chronic conditions, for both the health care practitioner and the for practitioner outreach to the child/family. In controlled trials the researchers found a significant positive influence of automatic reminders to families with children who have the diagnoses of asthma and attention deficit hyperactivity disorder (ADHD) were found to improve guideline adherence (Ferris 2009).

In a pediatric population, the use of screening and surveillance tools is an ongoing process as the healthcare professional monitors developmental changes. Online access to the multiple tools required for assessment as the child matures promotes the likelihood the screening will be performed. Linking to a central site such as is available from the University of Washington Medical Center's website, delivers routine screening as well as advanced screening tools in an efficient manner for the parent and health care professional (http://depts.washington.edu/ dbpeds/Screening%20Tools/ScreeningTools.html). Shared findings from screening with the family and entire care team assist coordination and goal prioritization in with a patient-centered focus.

One of the newest uses of technology supporting coordination is tracking engagement. Monitoring the child's engagement with health services is not limited to managed care entities who typically use claims data to compose an episode of care. Technology is available to track appointment adherence across multiple clinic and hospital visits. This is useful information for health providers who are part of an integrated delivery system or accountable care organization and are trying to effect children with chronic disease or frequent hospitalizations or emergency room use. One such example is Miami Children's Hospital, who utilizes a PatientPoint Tracker system as a population management tool. They have seen an improvement in patient engagement as families learn that the whole system is supporting visit attendance and continuity of care across the medical home and specialty providers (Leventhal 2013). Using the system not only ensures completion of needed testing or services at a visit but has improved the family experience, another important facet of overall compliance and care coordination.

References

Antonelli, R. (2013). *Empowering pediatric care coordination through technology*. Whitepaper.
Chase, D. (2012). Patient engagement is the blockbuster drug of the century. Retrieved from http://www.forbes.com/sites/davechase/2012/09/09/patient-engagement-is-the-blockbuster-drug-of-the-century
Ferris, T. (2009). *Improving pediatric safety and quality with healthcare information technology—final report. (Prepared by the Massachusetts General Hospital under Grant No. R01 HS 015002)*. Rockville, MD: Agency for Healthcare Research and Quality. Retrieved from http://healthit.ahrq.gov/sites/default/files/docs/activity/improving_pediatric_safety_and_quality_with_hit_2009_update_2.pdf
Frie, R. (2013). Technological changes can transform medicine by 2020: A conversation with the futurist Jim Carroll. *American Health & Drug Benefits, 6*(8), 510.
Glaser, J. (2013). Expanding patients role in their care. *Hospitals and Health Networks*. Retrieved from http://www.hhnmag.com/hhnmag/HHNDaily/HHNDailyDisplay.dhtml?id=7280003149
Health Information Technology for Economic and Clinical Health (HITECH) Act, Title XIII of Division A and Title IV of Division B of the American Recovery and Reinvestment Act of 2009 (ARRA), Pub. L. No. 111-5, 123 Stat. 226 (Feb. 17, 2009), *codified at* 42 U.S.C. §§300jj *et seq.*; §§17901 *et seq.* (2009). Retrieved from http://www.healthit.gov/policy-researchers-implementers/hitech-act-0
Leventhal, R. (2013). Keeping track of patients across the care continuum at Miami children's. *Healthcare Informatics*. Retrieved from: http://www.healthcare-informatics.com/article/keeping-track-patients-across-care-continuum-miami-children-s
Teich, J. (2013). Providers must rely on HIT to optimize care coordination. *Executive Insight*. Retrieved from http://inorderbyelseiver.com/2013/06/providers-must-rely-on-hit-to-optimize-care-coordination/
The National Alliance for Health Information Technology (2008). *Report to the office of the national coordinator for health information technology on defining key health information technology terms*. Washington, D.C.: Department of Health and Human Services. Retrieved from http://www.nacua.org/documents/HealthInfoTechTerms.pdf
Roper, R., Anderson, K., March, C., & Flemming, A. (2013). Health IT enabled quality measurement: Perspectives and practical guidance. Rockville, MD: Agency for Healthcare Research and Quality. Publication No. 13-0059-EF
Stricker, P. (2013). Supporting transitions of care with technology. *CMSA Today*. Retrieved from http://www.naylornetwork.com/cmsatoday/articles/index.asp?aid=229952&issueID=30156

Part III
Looking Ahead

Chapter 10
Future Directions in Case Management and Care Coordination

10.1 Influence and Trends

Care Coordination is an expanding field thanks in part to health care reform as well as evidence based studies indicating improvement in clinical outcomes of children as well as cost efficiencies. One example is Rhode Island's Pediatric Practice Enhancement Project, which used parent partners to assist families with children with special healthcare needs in service coordination, resulting in a decreased in admissions within their target group (Silow-Carroll 2009). The Community-based Pediatric Enhanced Care Program provided through Brenner Children's Hospital is another example of successful community-based care coordination for families of children with complex conditions making a difference for families (Murphy et al. 2012). Care coordination's use of scheduling assistance across specialties and compilation of resources will continue to be a strong foundational element of successful care coordination (Taylor et al. 2013). Texas Children's Health Plan in Houston, Texas, has been able to achieve statistically significant results in cost and admission reduction through utilizing embedded case managers to provide care coordination services to vulnerable children seen in high volume primary care offices (Treadwell 2014). Another example of cost savings is at Boston Children's Hospital. Their Community Asthma Initiative conducted a cost analysis for their program realizing an adjusted net present value savings from decreased emergency room visits and decreased admissions of $83,863 for 102 patients (Bhaumik et al. 2013).

Transition programs as seen in the Adolescent Health Transition Project of the University of Washington (http://depts.washington.edu/healthtr) are also expected to be on the rise. The Washington program site provides not only resources and support to families in their area, but offers open source forms, checklists, and processes to families and healthcare professionals in establishing solid transition programs that respect the growing autonomy of the adolescent. A similar resource to support the growing programming recognizing the importance of providing a

© The Author(s) 2015
J. Treadwell et al., *Case Management and Care Coordination*,
SpringerBriefs in Child Health, DOI 10.1007/978-3-319-07224-1_10

smooth transition to adult care is the national Center for Health Care Transition Improvement (http://www.gottransition.org/) organization which has resource toolkits for both families and health care providers.

Expansion of the Association of Maternal Child Health Programs (AMCHP) is another sign of growing innovation in the area of care coordination. The Oregon Care Coordination Program (CaCoon) is designated as a promising practice through the AMCHP Innovation Station (http://www.amchp.org). The Oregon program fosters face-to-face contact with families of children with special healthcare needs. During 2012, 1,836 children received 8,979 visits from CaCoon nurses. Children involved in this program had a 10 % reduction in hospitalizations during 2010 over the prior year. In addition to the impact they have made for families in Oregon, this program has developed a program manual and assessment tools as well as webinar training available to sites/families across the nation. Funding from Health Resources Services and Administration (HRSA) is in the middle of their five-year cycle, encouraging states to pursue studies to uncover improved ways to support children with special health care needs through case management and care coordination efforts. The Medical Home Implementation for Children with Special Healthcare Needs grants have provided technical assistance and funding to address expansion of medical homes (care coordination being one of the six medical home domains). HRSA grant activity requires communication and spread of coordination ideas across the state. Ideas, run through quick cycle improvement, test processes thought to be helpful. An example in Texas is use of a Care Ambassador approach to engage adolescents with diabetes in their ongoing appointment and testing needs supporting care coordination and self-management skill development. These grant-funded sites are important for the future as each state shares its innovation with sites across the nation encouraging replication or modification which will influence future best practice for care coordination.

Another future change will include certification requirements for case managers as opposed to the existing model of preference for certification. This will establish consumer protections around the knowledge and capabilities of the professional providing services and legislative definitions and parameters for service expectations and outcomes. Development of additional payment for case management services, increased use of technology as part of care coordination delivery funded through public-private partnerships, creation of fellowships to increase professionalism, research into the efficacy of new case management and care coordination models, will also be in effect. Increased use of Accountable Care Organizations (ACO) and Medical Homes as entities providing care coordination will increase to impact emergency room expense. The outcomes of that family-centered support and results of coordination should be seen in a rise of ambulatory care with emergency room use diminished.

The advent of Health Insurance Exchanges and the availability of healthcare coverage to individuals previously uninsured open the potential consumer base for care coordination. Another important facet of the Affordable Care Act is removal of lifetime limits, something extremely important to families of children with significant disabilities. This additional focus on care coordination will play into requirement for professional licensure, national certification and continuing education to ensure Americans are receiving a consistent level of professional capability and protection. The inclusion of care coordination as a need and expectation of insurance coverage also necessitates payment from commercial insurers in addition to the Centers for Medicaid and Medicare Services payment for care coordination of Medicare recipients.

Defined payment for care coordination services results in requirements of measurement and accountability. Care coordination as a component in Accountable Care Organizations (ACO) will define its product through these quality measurements. Pediatric Demonstration Projects occurring between 2012 and 2016 will identify how ACO's specifically focused on children will provide care for children enrolled in Medicaid and Children's Health Insurance Programs. Findings from these demonstration sites will inform structure of pediatric ACO's and move the payment and processes into the commercial systems. One of the known inclusions in these pilot sites is included behavioral health therapies in pediatric health homes. This role of psychiatry features both verbal and in-person on demand consultations for behavioral health issues (Martini and Houston 2013). Under this model of health service delivery, children will have greater access to behavioral health coordination with family focused coordination and communication of behavioral and physical health services.

> Tips for Parents: Co-located or professional associations between primary care and behavioral health teams should be available to your child. Ask your primary care provider what arrangements are in place within their practice.

> Tips for Health Care Professionals: There will be a challenge to move from autonomous practice to team communication behaviors. Ensuring access to psychiatry and social workers as well as development of communication and referral protocols are important.

Not surprisingly, use of lean strategies by case managers will be increasingly facilitated by managed care entities seeking to support improvements in population health. Using the quality initiative of lean and six sigma, will engage teams in finding efficiencies in processes to improve clinical and financial outcomes. One of the areas of lean review will be how to deal with children who have multiple health services use events for diagnoses categorized as potentially preventable. Potentially preventable emergency room visits, admissions and readmissions will play an important role to health plans and ACO's as well as hospitals as there is likelihood of a diminished or absent payment for health services deemed preventable. To give some context to this issue, in 2010, the United States had 1,85,000 potentially preventable hospitalizations (Torio et al. 2013). To reduce these events, care coordination will be at the lead, performing post-discharge medication reconciliation and establishing follow up visits with the child's care team to prevent readmission and reviewing barriers for individualized action in cases of readmission. Action to impact potentially preventable emergency room admissions includes active outreach to engage patients with care gaps of unfilled prescriptions or missed physician appointments, using motivational interviewing techniques to produce a call to action for chronic disease monitoring and preventive care.

10.2 Future Technology

Families and practitioners have an appetite for increased technology, to enhance communication, latest treatment information and access to care. Specifically in the field of tele-health engagement, services will be expanding in an effort to provide family centered, coordinated care. Existing telemedicine delivery in behavioral health therapies and tele-dermatology services will move to chronic condition self-management and engagement of asthma and diabetes for both office visits and monitoring. Use of innovative technology to facilitate patient engagement can be exampled in the GeckoCap (http://www.geckocap.com/). The GeckoCap uses Bluetooth technology and an embedded mobile application in an inhaler cap to send alerts, monitors use, and delivers incentives to children for compliant use. The result is self-management learning by the child as well as inclusion of the family/physician through enabling remote monitoring capability. Increasing engagement links directly to improved shared-decisions making where families will be able to look at alternative treatment and network.

An expansion of intuitive web-based internet sites integrating wellness, disease management and educational videos and interactive programs will be developed and used by care coordination teams to promote engagement and self-management as well as online support group expansion and personalized messaging. For example, the National Center for Medical Home Implementation has created more than 70 youtube videos developed by parent partner and physicians informing on the core components of medical homes (2013). Similarly, this same organization has employed an e-newsletter to inform the public of training events, advancements and new resources.

Families and health care providers will increasingly share best practice protocols, email exchanges and text communications. In one effort, Verizon Communications is working in conjunction with health care professionals to develop a partnership exploring how low-cost wireless technology like texting can be used to improve communication between patients and physicians (Antonelli and Ostrovsky, 2013). (http://responsibility.verizon.com/healthcare/childrens-health-fund.) The care team and family will utilize a shared care plan viewable on the online patient health record that will also display claim utilization, medication refill experience and patient preferences. Professionals will utilize predictive modeling to focus case managers and care coordination teams to prioritize contacts and will incorporate disease registries into both outreach and outcomes monitoring. The complete and searchable nature of health information exchanges will assist families in connections across specialists enabling accurate synopsis of health information without repeating forms or narratives of a child's health experience. This will promote earlier diagnosis and treatment across co-morbid states. I-pad or tablet technology use by care coordination team members will be used to increase the efficiency of documentation or additionally be used for face-to-face education and teleconferencing.

> Tips for Parents: Families can access guidelines from the Web. To ensure you are reviewing sound materials you may want to reference the National Guideline Clearinghouse (www.guideline.gov), the W.K. Kellogg Health Science Library (www.library.dal.ca/Kellogg), or sites of specialty organizations like the American Academy of Pediatrics (www.aap.org), and the American Academy of Child and Adolescent Psychiatry (www.aacap.org).

> Tips for Healthcare Professionals: Utilizing pathways, guidelines and standards of care enhances clear communication across the care team. Clear understanding of the chosen protocols and goals reduces care fragmentation and decreases service duplication. The case manager and care team will have greater success in initiating and monitoring a plan developed through shared decision-making, inclusive of a evidenced-based foundation.

Applications to expand communication ability for non-verbal children or improve mobilization is also expected to increase. For example SPEAK all! has been reported by Purdue University to improve the ability for children with autism to communicate through associated images (http://www.purdue.edu/newsroom/releases/2013/Q2/apps-may-open-communication-door-for-children,-families-affected-by-severe,-non-verbal-autism.html). This application is available for free through iTunes and is representative of technology innovation that can allow children to become more participate in their own care planning by making their needs and preferences known. Removing barriers to care, identified by the family and healthcare team such as communication issues, is an optimal use of technology. Another type of communication using technology is seen in chronic condition management where there is often call for reminders of compliance. Reminder systems such as *Voice Shot* (http://www.voiceshot.com/public/patientreminder.asp?ref=ARMed_patient+reminder+systems) function as a reminder for medications that can foster compliance and independence in teens. Akron Children's hospital recognized a need for use of this type of technology in children after bone marrow transplant. Non-adherence to medication impacts the rejection after transplant increases overall costs. Systems supporting engagement and adherence to jointly developed plans of care help families integrate the electronic medical record for monitoring and provide an on-demand education communication capability.

Case management software, utilized by the care management teams currently contains clinical support tools and algorithms which support comprehensive assessments and care planning. Popular guidelines incorporated into case management software applications today include Interqual and Milliman. These tools will be further enhanced to include the latest guidelines and predictive capabilities.

10.3 Medical Homes and Support Groups

The rework of the delivery system to invest in patient-centered medical homes will increase the need for ambulatory care coordination. The past reluctance of primary care providers to handle complex cases should ease as provision of access incorporated into Accountable Care Organizations will encourage practitioners to spend more time with patients instead of the current pay by visit mentality. While the concentration of pediatric subspecialties will likely continue in urban locations, increasing links to community providers will be delivered through technology-supported consultations to support delivery of services closest to the child's home whenever possible. Telemedicine has been shown to reduce pediatric medication errors in rural emergency departments, a benefit for coordination across the continuum of care (http://www.ucdmc.ucdavis.edu/publish/news/pediatrics/8365).

Incorporation of the consumer will be extremely important with changing models of delivery and benefits. Both health plans and medical homes will establish and/or expand consumer advisory panels that are heavily involved in understanding the patient/family experience in receiving healthcare. Support groups for families have been reported to be successful in creating communication of usable information and a variant perspective than that obtained from the healthcare community. An example of use of social support networks, believed to be a growing vehicle for families described by Janvier et al. (2012) indicated families involved in support groups seemed able to celebrate small achievements and have hopes and expectations of the provider community due to what they have learned through this social engagement. Care coordination teams will need to be able to respond and support the family autonomy and requests resulting from acquired knowledge of choices and treatments.

10.4 Recommendations and Strategies for the Future

Case management fellowships will increase in academic centers to encourage case managers to enter the care coordination field specific to the special needs child, further developing the discipline. These fellowship opportunities will give case managers a solid foundation in integrated case management. The importance of transitions of care should translate to an increased emphasis on transitioning adolescents to adult care and children between care settings as required components of continuing education. Each state has varying continuing education requirements however, the case management certification adds specific continuing education requirement applicable to the practice of case management. Development of competency-based requirements for positions on the care coordination team will include skill sets for case managers, navigators/community health workers/parent partners. High on that list of competencies will be motivational interviewing and communication skills, followed closely by demonstration of an understanding of the current legislative, regulatory, and benefit frameworks for programs. The changing landscape for insurance coverage and coordination standards will require continual attention for employers of care coordination teams.

Evidence based practice will continue to grow influenced by continuing research, funding requirements favoring established evidenced-based programming, and protocol development by health plans, professional societies, insurers and advocacy groups partnering to develop efficiencies and quality improvements to meet the requirements for our changing delivery system.

Online training and post graduate degrees are another expanding future opportunity for case management. Currently the University of Alabama offers Case Management/Leadership as a Master's degree nursing program. Undergraduate programs are now including case management into undergraduate curriculums as well as exampled by Idaho State University. The Maternal Child Health Bureau is developing a standardized pediatric care coordination curriculum and other entities such as the Case Management Society of America is developing online curriculum for pediatric assessments and care planning.

10.5 Conclusion

Family centered care puts forth that health services will be accessible, coordinated, culturally effective, compassionate and continuous providing children and families a voice in care delivery and choice of treatment. Movement toward that goal is actively being pursued by advocacy organizations, accrediting entities, credentialing organizations, managed care companies and Accountable Care Organizations. Addressing the needs of vulnerable populations require care coordination services to facilitate the health care professional plan of care in the context of the family needs, desires and preferences. Coordinated care delivery, supported by a professional team of case managers, navigators, parent partners and support staff are best suited to facilitate positive outcomes and accept the change in healthcare reimbursement for value.

Improved care coordination, utilizing technology to enhance communication between all care professionals and the family will transform healthcare to achieve the quality focus consumers are demanding. Case management and care coordination are an integral part of team-based care that is necessary to achieve this value-based care. The 2009/2010 National Survey of Children with Special Healthcare Needs indicated that 11.2 million children (ages 0–17) living in the United States have a special healthcare need (2013). There is reason to believe that number will expand as access to insurance coverage increases and technology continues to improve interventions. Long-term acute care and skilled nursing centers are very limited for pediatric patients, making the need for in-home coordination to meet the child's needs essential (Greene 2012). Families need support in managing their conditions and in facilitating communication between healthcare professionals. Case management and care coordination comes to these newer models of care armed with the skills of interprofessional collaboration to support effective use of teams.

The success of case management and care coordination will be documented through outcomes measurement. Outcomes are an integral part of the overall accountability and quality improvement documentation expressing the value proposition of case management. The goals set by the care team (with the family as an integral part of that team) are the yardstick for measurement. Monitoring of the plan's effectiveness throughout the relationship assists the team in knowing when to change strategies or add/modify services in order to reach the designated and prioritized goals for the child/family.

References

Antonelli, R., & Ostrovsky, A. (2013, June). *Empowering Care Coordination with Technology: Opportunities to Transform Pediatric Care Delivery*. Verizon Foundation Whitepaper. Retrieved from http://responsibility.verizon.com/assets/docs/BCH-VZF-Care-Coordination-White-Paper-June-2013.pdf.

Bhaumik, U., Norris, K., Gisele, C., Walker, S., Sommer, S., Chan, E., & et al. (2013, April). A cost analysis for a community-based case management intervention program for pediatric asthma. *Journal of Asthma, 50*(3), 310.

Greene, D. (2012). The health care home model: primary health care meeting public health goals. *American Journal of Public Health, 102*, 1096–1103. doi:10.2105/AJPH.2011. Retrieved from http://insurancenewsnet.com/oarticle/2012/06/01/the-health-care-home-model-primary-health-care-meeting-public-health-goals-%5Bame-a-344579.html.

Janvier, A., Farlow, B., & Wilfond, B. (2012). The experience of families of children with trisomy 13 and 18 in social netwiorks. *Pediatrics, 130*, 293–298. doi:10.1542/peds.2012-0151. Retrieved from http://pediatrics.aappublications.org/content/early/2012/07/18/peds.2012-0151.full.pdf+html.

Martini, R., & Houston, M. (2013, March). ACO's and CAPs: Preparing for the impact of healthcare reform on child and adolescent psychiatry practice. American Academy of Child and Adolescent Psychiatry. Retrieved from http://www.aacap.org/App_Themes/AACAP/Docs/homepage/2013/preparing_for_healthcare_reform_201303.pdf.

Murphy, J., Kobayashi, D., Golden, S., & Nageswaran, S. (2012). Rural and non-rural differences in the system of care for children with complex chronic conditions. *Pediatrics, 51*(5), 498–503. doi:10.1177/0009922812436884. Retrieved from http://cpj.sagepub.com/content/51/5/498.

National Center for Medical Home Implementation. (2013). *A Retrospective Look at Programs and Initiatives Toward Family-Centered Medical Home for Every Child and Youth*. Maternal and Child Health Bureau grant U43MC09134. Retrieved from http://www.medicalhomeinfo.org/downloads/pdfs/NCMHI%20Retrospective_FINAL_July2013.pdf.

Policy memorandum Department of Defense on patient centered medical homes. (2009, Sep 18). Retrieved from http://www.bethesda.med.navy.mil/patient/health_care/medical_services/internal_medicine/PCMH%20Policy%20Memo%20-%20signed.pdf.

Shoemaker, MD, S. (2010, March). Commentary: Health care payment reform and academic medicine: Threat or opportunity? *Academic Medicine*.

Silow-Carroll, S. (2009). Rhode Island's pediatric practice enhancement project: Parents helping parents and practitioners, 20 pp. NY: Common wealth Fund. http://www.commonwealthfund.

org/~/media/Files/Publications/Case%20Study/2010/Jan/1361_SilowCarroll_Rhode_Island_ PPEP_case_study.pdf

Silow-Carroll, S., & Hagelow, G. (2011). Effective pediatric case management. *Care Management, 17*, 7–13. Retrieved from http://nursing.msu.edu/Images_Docs/CE_Images/ CasePresentations/GwenFosse.pdf.

Taylor, A., Lizzi, M., Marx, A., Chilkatowsky, M., Trachtenberg, S., & Ogle, S. (2013). Implementing a care coordination program for children with special healthcare needs: partnering with families and providers. *Journal of Healthcare Quality, 35*(5), 70–77.

The Institute of Medicine, Committee on Quality of Health Care In America. *Crossing the Quality Chasm.* Washington, D.C. National Academy Press. 2001.

Torio, C., Elixhauser, A., & Andrews, R. (2013). Trends in Potentially Preventable Hospital Admissions among Adults and Children,2005–2010. Healthcare Cost and Utilization Project, Agency for Healthcare Research and Quality. Statistical Brief #151. Retrieved from http:// www.hcup-us.ahrq.gov/reports/statbriefs/sb151.pdf.

Treadwell, J. (2014, March/April) Collaborating for Care: Initial experience of embedded case managers across five medical homes. *Professional Case Management, 19*(2), 86–92.

UC Davis Health System Department of Pediatrics. *Telemedicine reduces pediatric medication errors in rural emergency departments.* Retrieved from http://www.ucdmc.ucdavis.edu/ publish/news/pediatrics/8365.

Index

© The Author(s) 2015
J. Treadwell et al., *Case Management and Care Coordination*,
SpringerBriefs in Child Health, DOI 10.1007/978-3-319-07224-1

Printed in the United States
By Bookmasters

Printed in the United States
By Bookmasters